Journal of Vascular Research

Founded 1964 as 'Angiologica' by M. Comèl and L. Laszt (1964–1973)
continued as 'Blood Vessels' by J.A. Bevan (1974–1991)

KARGER

Printed in Denmark
by SVFs Fællestrykkeri, Aarhus

Guidelines for Authors

Journal of Vascular Research

Journal of Vascular Research publishes manuscripts of scientific excellence in vascular and lymphatic biology, physiology and pathophysiology. The scope of the journal covers a broad spectrum of vascular and lymphatic research, including vascular structure, vascular function, haemodynamics, mechanics, cell signalling, intercellular communication, growth and differentiation. Papers employing cellular, biophysical and molecular techniques, as well as more classical approaches are welcomed. Manuscripts may be in the form of research papers, reviews, rapid communications and correspondence.

Submission
Only original manuscripts written in English are considered. Research papers and reviews should not normally be more than 10 printed pages in length including illustrations and references (6,460 characters per page). Authors wishing to submit a review should contact the Editors in advance. Rapid communications should not exceed 3 printed pages. Correspondence and Commentary should be brief. Manuscripts should be sent to:

Main Editor: Prof. Michael J. Mulvany
Department of Pharmacology
University of Aarhus
University Park 240
DK–8000 Aarhus C
Denmark
Tel. + 45 8942 1726
Fax + 45 8612 8804

except for manuscripts from North America, which should be sent to:

Associate Editor: Dr. Gary K. Owens
Department of Physiology
University of Virginia, Box 449
1300 Jefferson Park Avenue
Charlottesville, VA 22908
USA
Tel. + 1 804 924 2652 or 0524
Fax + 1 804 982 0055

To facilitate a rapid review process, authors are asked to supply their telephone and fax numbers.

Manuscripts, including photocopies of line drawings, should be submitted in quadruplicate, typewritten double-spaced on one side of the paper, 10 characters per inch, with a margin not less than 25 mm on each side. Two photographs of line-drawings and four copies of micrographs should be supplied on glossy paper.

Conditions
All manuscripts are subject to editorial review. Manuscripts are received with the explicit understanding that they are not under simultaneous consideration by any other publication. Submission of an article for publication implies the transfer of the copyright from the author to the publisher upon acceptance. Accepted papers become the permanent property of 'Journal of Vascular Research' and may not be reproduced by any means, in whole or in part, without the written consent of the publisher. It is the author's responsibility to obtain permission to reproduce illustrations, tables, etc. from other publications.

Arrangement of Research papers
Manuscript organization: Manuscripts should include, in sequence and on separate pages: title and authors, address, running title and acknowledgment of support; abstract and key words; introduction; methods; results; discussion; acknowledgments; references; tables; figures. The normal maximum length is 10 printed pages (including tables, illustrations and references), one printed page containing 6,460 letters, spaces included.

Title page: The first page of each paper should indicate the title (main title underlined), the authors' names, and the institute where the work was conducted. A short title for use as running head is also required.

Full address: The exact postal address complete with postal code must be given at the bottom of the title page. Please also supply phone and fax numbers, as well as your e-mail address.

Key words: For indexing purposes, a list of 3–10 key words in English is essential. Consult previous numbers of Journal of Vascular Research for suitable entries.

Abstract: Each paper needs an abstract of up to 200 words.

Style: All measurements should normally be in SI units. Blood pressure may be given in mm Hg. Use generic names of drugs. Avoid jargon, euphemisms and abbreviations.

Small type: Paragraphs which can or must be set in smaller type (case histories, test methods, etc.) should be indicated with a 'p' (petit) in the margin on the left-hand side.

Footnotes: Acknowledgment of support is printed as a footnote to the title. Other footnotes should be avoided. When essential, they are numbered consecutively and typed at the foot of the appropriate page.

Tables and illustrations: Tables and illustrations (both numbered in Arabic numerals) should be prepared on separate sheets. Tables require a heading and figures a legend, also prepared on a separate sheet. For the reproduction of illustrations, only good drawings and original photographs can be accepted; negatives or photocopies cannot be used. Due to technical reasons, figures with a screen background should not be submitted. When possible, group several illustrations on one block for reproduction (max. size 181 × 223 mm) or provide crop marks. On the back of each illustration, indicate its number, the author's name, and 'top' with a soft pencil.

Color illustrations: Up to 6 color illustrations per page can be integrated with the text at the reduced price of CHF 600.– / USD 545.00 per page. Color illustrations are reproduced at the author's expense.

References: In the text identify references by Arabic numerals [in square brackets]. Material submitted for publication but not yet accepted should be noted as 'unpublished data' and not be included in the reference list. The list of references should include only those publications which are cited in the text. Do not alphabetize; number references in the order in which they are first mentioned in the text. The surnames of the authors followed by initials should be given. There should be no punctuation other than a comma to separate the authors. Cite all authors, 'et al' is not sufficient. Abbreviate journal names according to the Index Medicus system. (Also see International Committee of Medical Journal Editors: Uniform requirements for manuscripts submitted to biomedical journals. Br Med J 1988;296:401–405.)

Examples
(a) Papers published in periodicals: Shirahase H, Fujiwara M, Usui H, Kurahashi K: A possible role of thromboxane A_2 in endothelium in maintaining resting tone and producing contractile response to acetylcholine and arachidonic acid in canine cerebral arteries. Blood Vessels 1987;24:117–119.
(b) Monographs: Matthews DE, Farewell VT: Using and Understanding Medical Statistics, ed 3, revised. Basel, Karger, 1996.
(c) Edited books: Duling BR, Sleek GE: Mechanical aspects of endothelial cell–smooth muscle cell interactions in resistance vessels; in Bevan JA, Majewski H, Maxwell RH, Story DF (eds): Vascular Neuroeffector Mechanisms. Oxford, IRL Press, 1988, pp 23–30.

Further details: Authors may consult our leaflet 'Rules for the Preparation of Manuscripts', available on request from the Publisher, S. Karger AG, P.O. Box, CH–4009 Basel (Switzerland).

Rapid communication
Manuscripts intended for rapid communication must present new findings of sufficient importance to justify their accelerated acceptance. They should follow the general arrangement of research papers. No abstracts or introduction is required, but the first paragraph should include the reason for the study and the main findings. The general format for Research Papers should be followed, but they should not be more than three printed pages in length (including figures, tables and references). Proofs are checked by the Main Editor and not sent to the authors. Review will be rapid, and once accepted, the paper will be included in the next planned issue.

Reviews
Reviews concerned with topics in vascular research of current interest will be welcomed. Potential authors are asked to check first with the Editors to avoid clashes with other pending reviews. All reviews will be subjected to normal critical peer refereeing.

Correspondence
Letters to the Editor concerning articles published in Journal of Vascular Research may be submitted for publication. If accepted, the authors of the articles concerned will be given the opportunity to reply.

Commentary
Comments concerning current topics of interest in vascular science will be considered for publication by the Editors. They should not be more than one printed page.

Page charges
Authors are charged CHF 75.– / USD 53.00 per printed page. 1 printed page is equal to approximately 2 manuscript pages. Where an author is unable to pay these charges, they may be waived at the discretion of the Editors.

Galley proofs
Unless indicated otherwise, galley proofs are sent to the first-named author and should be returned with the least possible delay. Alterations made in galley proofs, other than the correction of printer's errors, are charged to the author. No page proofs are supplied.

Reprints
Order forms and a price list are sent with the galley proofs. Orders submitted after the issue is printed are subject to considerably higher prices. Allow five weeks from date of publication for delivery of reprints.

KARGER
E-Mail karger@karger.ch
Fax + 41 61 306 12 34
http://www.karger.ch

The Guidelines for Authors are available at:
http://www.karger.ch/journals/jvr/jvrinst.htm

Journal of Vascular Research

General Information

Publication data: 'Journal of Vascular Research' is published 6 times annually. Volume 34 with 6 issues appears in 1997.

Subscription rates: Subscriptions run for a full calendar year. Prices are given per volume.
Personal subscription:
Subscription + postage and handling
CHF 94.50 + CHF 23.50 Europe
CHF 94.50 + CHF 35.50 Overseas
USD 72.60 + USD 23.50
(Must be in the name of, billed to, and paid by an individual. Order must be marked 'personal subscription'.)
Institutional subscription:
Subscription + postage and handling
CHF 626.– + CHF 29.40 Europe
CHF 626.– + CHF 44.40 Overseas
USD 522.00 + USD 29.40
Airmail postage: CHF 36.–, USD 30.00.
(Extra per volume.)

Microforms: Please direct all enquiries and orders to: University Microfilms Inc.
300 North Zeeb Road, P.O. Box 1346
Ann Arbor, MI 48106-1346 (USA)

Subscription orders: Orders can be placed at agencies, bookstores, directly with the Publisher
S. Karger AG, P.O. Box,
CH–4009 Basel (Switzerland)
or with any of the following distributors:
Deutschland: S. Karger GmbH, Postfach
D–79095 Freiburg
France: Librairie Luginbühl
36, bd de Latour-Maubourg, F–75007 Paris
Great Britain, Ireland: S. Karger Publishers
11 Ravenscroft Road
Beckenham, Kent BR3 4TP
USA: S. Karger Publishers, Inc.
26 West Avon Road, P.O. Box 529
Farmington, CT 06085
India, Bangladesh, Sri Lanka:
S. Karger India Subscription Agency
B–5/132 Safdarjung Enclave
New Delhi-110029
Japan: Katakura Libri, Inc.
Take 1 Bldg, 2nd Floor, 4-5-7 Yushima
Bunkyo-ku, Tokyo 113

Change of address: Both old and new address should be sent to the subscription source.

Single issues and back volumes: Information can be obtained through the Publisher.

Advertising: Correspondence and rate requests should be addressed to the Publisher.

Bibliographic indices: This journal is regularly listed in bibliographic services, including *Current Contents®*, Index Medicus, Reference Update, Biological Abstracts.

Copying: This journal has been registered with the Copyright Clearance Center (CCC), as indicated by the code appearing on the first page of each article.
For readers in the US, this code signals consent for copying of articles for personal or internal use, or for the personal or internal use of specific clients, provided that the stated fee is paid per copy directly to
Copyright Clearance Center Inc.
222 Rosewood Drive
Danvers, MA 01923 (USA)
A copy of the first page of the article must accompany payment. Consent does not extend to copying for general distribution, for promotion, for creating new works, or for resale. In these cases, specific written permission must be obtained from the copyright owner,
S. Karger AG,
P.O. Box, CH–4009 Basel (Switzerland).

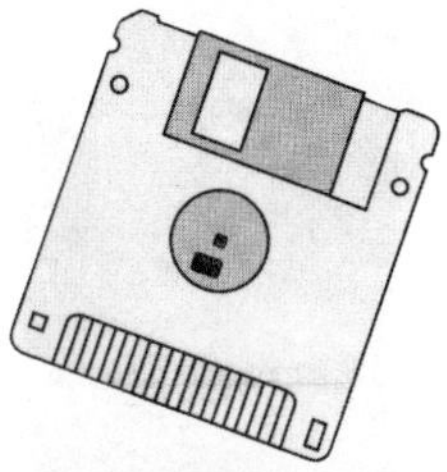

Guidelines for Disk Submission

Karger Publishers welcomes the submission of manuscripts on disk.
Please observe the 'Guidelines for Authors' as well as the following guidelines:

Technical Data
Storage medium is a 3.5- or 5.25-inch disk. **The preferred word processing package is Word for Windows®.** Other commonly used PC text programs are also accepted, as well as ASCII formats. MacIntosh® is also acceptable. However **1.44 MB HD** in ASCII is preferred.

Handling
All manuscripts accepted for Karger publications are subject to copy-editing. It is therefore essential that you send us a **double-spaced printout** of your manuscript which exactly matches the disk.
Any subsequent revised versions should be clearly marked as such, both on the disk and on the manuscript.
The copy-edited manuscript and the disk will be returned to you along with the galley proofs. Please be sure to **check the galleys against the manuscript** in which changes introduced by the copy-editor and/or questions will be marked.
Please **label** your disk with (a) the title of the journal or book for which it is submitted, (b) a short version of the paper title, (c) your name, (d) the software and hardware used and (e) the file names contained.
Do not place more than one article in a file.

Text Arrangement
Please follow the general rules about style given in the 'Guidelines for Authors' or 'Rules for the Preparation of Manuscripts'.
Be sure to use the same type style for headings of the same ranking throughout the text. Be consistent and stick to the same work pattern throughout the manuscript.
Do not use automatic page numbering. Number the pages by hand.
Text and headings should be ranged left throughout, without word breaks. **Do not center, space, or use block letters** for text and headings (except for abbreviations). Do not split words (neither by hand nor automatically). **Do not use indentations** anywhere in the manuscript, including the references.
To mark the beginning of a paragraph, leave one blank line between paragraphs. Do not use a hyphenating program. Use the possibilities of your text program to emphasize text parts, e.g. **Bold,** *Italic,* $_{\text{Sub-}}$ and ^{Superscript}.
Insert one (and only one) space after each interpunctuation mark – e.g. at the end of sentences and with reference numbers, i.e. [22, 27, 35].
When using **special characters** not available on a standard keyboard (including Greek characters) please do so by a readily identifiable code, and use the same code throughout the manuscript. Supply a **complete list of the codes used** at the beginning of the text or include a 'Read-me-file'.
Do not use spaces in tables; use the tabulator.
Operation data within tables (e.g. 15.1 ± 7.23) should be formatted in one column, not split into two.
Illustrations and mathematical formulae will be handled conventionally.

KARGER

E-Mail karger@karger.ch
Fax + 41 61 306 12 34
http://www.karger.ch

The Journal Home Page is available at:
http://www.karger.ch/journals/jvr/jvrdes.htm

Journal of Vascular Research

7th Symposium on Mechanisms of Vasodilatation

Maastricht, The Netherlands
July 6–9, 1997

KARGER

Journal of Vascular Research
Vol. 34, Supplement 1, 1997

Organizing Committee

P.M. Vanhoutte, Courbevoie
C.M. Boulanger, Paris
J.G.R. De Mey, Maastricht
N.A. Flavahan, Baltimore
R.S. Reneman, Maastricht
H.A.J. Struijker Boudier, Maastricht

Scientific Committee

J.A. Angus, Parkville
J.A. Bevan, Burlington
D.F. Bohr, Ann Arbor
G. Burnstock, London
R. Busse, Frankfurt am Main
R.A. Cohen, Boston
B. Duling, Charlottesville
J.E. Faber, Chapel Hill
E. Feigl, Seattle
B.B. Fredholm, Stockholm
R.F. Furchgott, Brooklyn
D.D. Heistad, Iowa City
Z.S. Katusic, Rochester
B.I. Lévy, Paris
T.F. Lüscher, Zürich
J.C. McGrath, Glasgow
G. Mancia, Monza
W. Martin, Glasgow
T. Masaki, Kyoto
V.M. Miller, Rochester
J.-V. Mombouli, Houston
S. Moncada, London
M.J. Mulvany, Aarhus
R.L. Prewitt, Norfolk
J.L. Reid, Glasgow
G. Rubanyi, Richmond
C.F. Sanchez-Ferrer, Madrid
V.B. Schini-Kerth, Frankfurt am Main
T. Scott-Burden, Houston
J.T. Shepherd, Rochester
A.P. Somlyo, Charlottesville
J.-C. Stoclet, Illkirch
A. Tedgui, Paris
N. Toda, Shiga
M. Tuncer, Ankara
J. Vane, London
S.F. Vatner, Southborough
T. Verbeuren, Suresnes
E.S. Vizi, Budapest

Sponsors

Institut de Recherches Internationales Servier (IRIS)
Cardiovascular Research Institute Maastricht (CARIM)

KARGER

S. Karger
Medical and Scientific Publishers
Basel · Freiburg · Paris · London
New York · New Delhi · Bangkok
Singapore · Tokyo · Sydney

Drug Dosage
The authors and the publisher have exerted every effort to ensure that drug selection and dosage set forth in this text are in accord with current recommendations and practice at the time of publication. However, in view of ongoing research, changes in government regulations, and the constant flow of information relating to drug therapy and drug reactions, the reader is urged to check the package insert for each drug for any change in indications and dosage and for added warnings and precautions. This is particularly important when the recommended agent is a new and/or infrequently employed drug.

P.O. Box, CH–4009 Basel (Switzerland)
Printed in Denmark by SVFs Fællestrykkeri, Aarhus
ISBN 3–8055–6543–7

J Vasc Res 1997;34(suppl 1):1-48

001

MUSCLE BLOOD FLOW IN CHRONIC COMPARTMENT SYNDROME. CONTINUOUS MEASUREMENT WITH LASER DOPPLER FLOWMETRY.

P. Abraham, G. Leftheriotis, J.L. Saumet.
Laboratoire de physiologie. C.H.U.. 49033 Angers cedex 01, France

Although largely used as a diagnostic criterion in chronic compartment syndrome, intracompartmental pressure measurements provide no direct information about the muscle blood flow disorder resulting from high tissue pressure. Continuous measurements of muscle blood flow with an implantable laser Doppler flowmeter probe and of intra compartment pressure were performed following exercise in 7 patients with compartment syndrome and 7 normal subjects. In compartment syndrome and in normal subjects respectively, compartmental pressure (mm Hg) was 74.1+/-4.4 and 24.2+/-3.4, one minute following exercise and decreased to 34.6+/-2.3 and 15.0+/-1.6 at 20 min (mean+/-SEM), muscle blood flow (Arb. Units) was 1.09+/-0.14 and 0.80+/-0.11 (N.S) 1 min following exercise and 0.41+/-0.11 and 0.27+/-0.04 (N.S) at the end of the recovery period. Although pressure showed a progressive decrease over time in both groups, muscle blood flow decreased sharply during the first minutes of recovery in normal subjects whereas in patients with compartment syndrome a delayed hyperemic peak was found muscle blood flow reaching 0.84+/-0.10 in compartment syndrome and 0.33+/-0.06 in normal subjects ($p<0.01$) at minute 9. Although individual differences were found on increased tissue pressure tolerance, a threshold can be found after which micro-circulation is altered though muscle blood flow does not cease. Laser Doppler flowmetry appears as an interesting technique for the study of the physiopathology and in the diagnosis of compartment syndrome.

002

MECHANISM OF NITRIC OXIDE PRODUCTION BY WINE POLYPHENOLS IN BOVINE AORTIC ENDOTHELIAL CELLS

E. Andriambeloson, J. Duarte, A. Kleschyov, J.C. Stoclet and R. Andriantsitohaina.
Laboratoire de Pharmacologie, URA CNRS 600, BP 24, F 67401 Illkirch-Cedex.

We have previously reported that some polyphenols contained in wine possess potent endothelium-dependent vasorelaxing activity. This effect results from enhanced synthesis of NO from the endothelium. We further studied the mechanisms by which polyphenolic extract stimulated the production of NO in cultured bovine aortic endothelial cells.

Changes in intracellular calcium in endothelial cells suspension were measured using the fluorescent indicator fura 2. Polyphenolic extract at a concentration at which it produced maximal endothelium-dependent vasorelaxing activity (0.01 g/l), elicited a transient increase in cytosolic calcium. This effect was abolished in calcium-free medium and in the presence of N-ethylmaleimide (100 µM), but not altered by pertussis toxin (600 ng/ml). This increase in cytosolic calcium was not affected by the NADPH-oxidase inhibitor, diphenyliodonium (10 µM) and by the cytochrome-P450 inhibitor, clotrimazole (10 µM) but was reduced by the combination of superoxide dismutase (100 U/ml) and catalase (100 U/ml). Furthermore, polyphenolic extract stimulated superoxide anion production of cultured endothelial cells determined by cytochrome C reduction assay. NO spin trapping and electron paramagnetic resonance studies showed that leucocyanidol, one of the wine polyphenols compounds produced an increase in NO levels in endothelial cells. This effect was abolished by the NO-synthase inhibitor, N^G-nitro-L-arginine methyl ester (300 µM)

It is concluded that wine polyphenols stimulate NO production via an influx of calcium from extracellular source. This effect involves a production of superoxide anion in cultured bovine aortic endothelial cells. The latter effect is mediated by a pertussis toxin-insensitive and NADPH-oxidase-independent mechanisms.

1018-1172/97/0347-0001$12.00/0

003

REDUCED NORADRENALINE-MEDIATED VASODILATATON AND β-ADRENOCEPTOR DENSITY IN THE BASILAR ARTERY DURING AGEING.

S.M. Arribas, *A.F. Dominiczak and J.C. McGrath.
CRI in Heart Failure, IBLS, *Department of Medicine and Therapeutics, Western Infirmary, University of Glasgow, UK.

The aim of the present study was to analyze in basilar arteries from young (4 month old) and old (12 month old) Wistar-Kyoto rats the possible alteration with age in β-adrenoceptor function and density. Segments were mounted on a wire myograph, normalized at 0.91_{100} and responses to agonists determined. For receptor localization, the arteries were stained with the fluorescent derivative of the β-agonist CGP-12177A (BODIPY-CGP) and visualized with Laser Scanning Confocal Microscopy (Odyssey, EX 488 nm, EM 515 nm). In 4 month old WKY rats, noradrenaline (1nM-30μM) produced concentation-dependent relaxations in basal conditions (n=4 rats). Propranolol (1 μM) induced vasoconstriction and in its presence noradrenaline induced concentration-dependent contractions. In 12 month old rats, noradrenaline produced no response or small concentration-dependent contractions (n=5 rats). BODIPY-CGP (10nM), revealed discrete clusters of binding localized in the media. No fluorescence was visualized in the endothelium. The intensity of fluorescence was significantly reduced in the presence of 1μM propranolol (average intensity 8±0.89 brightness/pixel; p<0.01 vs control) and unchanged by the α-adrenoceptor blocker prazosin. BODIPY-CGP fluorescence was significantly reduced in arteries from old rats (young, average intenstiy 53.7±4.5 brightness/pixel; old, average intensity 3.4±0.2 brightness/pixel; p<0.01 vs young). These results suggest that in the rat basilar artery there is : (1) an important β-adrenoceptor activity mediating vasodilatation, (2) this activity decreases during ageing and (3) these decrease might be due to reduction in SMC β-adrenoceptor density.

Supported by British Heart Foundation, MRC and Biomed.

004

COMPARATIVE STUDY OF NEURONAL ORGANIZATION OF LIMBIC MECHANISMS OF VASOMOTOR REGULATION

O.G.Baklavadjian
Orbeli Institute of Physiology Arm.Acad.Sciences, 22 Orbeli Br.Str., Yerevan 375028, Armenia

In anesthetized and immobilized cats it was shown that low-frequency (5 Hz) stimulation of most hypothalamic structures, ventral part of area 25 and of all nuclear regions of amygdala induced vasodilatation and arterial depressor reactions, while high-frequency (100 Hz) stimulation of the same areas evoked vasoconstriction and an obvious pressure response. Both frequencies of stimulation of some structures of posterior hypothalamus elicited pressure reactions only, while low- and high-frequency stimulation of a restricted area of anterior hypothalamus and dorsal regions of areas 25 and 24 of limbic cortex induced vasodilatation and depressor reaction. The observed three patterns of arterial blood pressure responses to low- and high-frequency stimulation of limbic structures are related to rigid connections of some hypothalamic and limbic cortex areas and flexible connections of divergent type polyeffectory neurons of some limbic structures with bulbo-spinal sympatho-activating and sympatho-inhibitory systems of vasomotor regulation.

In a series of microelectrophysiological investigation it was shown that single or train stimulation of different hypothalamic structures evoked monosynaptic activation of some antidromically identified bulbo-spinal neurons of dorsocaudal and ventrolateral sympatho-activating regions. Firing rate of some neurons is increased by high-frequency stimulation and depressed by low-frequency stimulation of the hypothalamus.

Possible neuronal organization of limbic mechanisms of vasomotor regulation are discussed.

005

EXPRESSION OF INDUCIBLE NITRIC OXIDE SYNTHASE IN ATHEROSCLEROTIC LESIONS OF CHOLESTEROL-FED RABBITS

D. Behr[2], A. Rupin[1], J.-N. Fabiani[2] et T.J. Verbeuren[1]
[1] Division of Angiology, SERVIER Research Institute, 92150 Suresnes, France; [2] Laboratoire d'étude des greffes et prothèses cardiaques, Hôpital Broussais, 75014 Paris, France

Evidence for a functional non-endothelial NO-synthase and an increased activity of guanylate cyclase have been reported in aortas of hypercholesterolemic rabbits [Verbeuren TJ et al. J Cardiovasc Pharmacol 1993;21:841-845; Rupin A et al. Brit J Pharmacol 1996;119:1233-1238].

To study the expression of inducible nitric oxide synthase (NOS-II) at different levels of the vascular tree, indirect immuno-fluorescence was performed on frozen tissue sections from New-Zealand white rabbits fed a 0.3% cholesterol diet for 45 weeks. Incubation of serial sections with monoclonal antibodies RAM-11 and HHF-35 respectively revealed the constant presence of numerous macrophages in the neo-intima but a variable infiltration of smooth muscle cells in the fibro-muscular cap of well-developed lesions of the thoracic and abdominal aortas, the coronary and pulmonary arteries. In contrast, lesions of the carotid and femoral arteries were sparse and rarely displayed a fibro-muscular cap. On adjacent sections of the thoracic and abdominal aortas, the coronary and pulmonary arteries, the NOS-II antibody revealed punctiform stainings in the neo-intima where macrophages have accumulated. A more diffuse but intense signal was found in the subendothelial layer and in the media. In contrast, no expression of NOS-II was detected in the carotid and femoral arteries, or in samples from control rabbits. The specificity of the anti-NOS-II antibody was assessed by western blot.

This study provides evidence for the expression of NOS-II in advanced arterial lesions of hypercholesterolemic rabbits and suggests its induction in different cell types such as macrophages and smooth muscle cells.

006

LACK OF BRADYKININ-INDUCED SMOOTH MUSCLE CELL HYPERPOLARIZATION DESPITE HETEROCELLULAR DYE COUPLING AND ENDOTHELIAL CELL HYPERPOLARIZATION IN PORCINE CILIARY ARTERY

J.-L. Bény, *P. Zhu, *I. O. Haefliger
Department of Zoology and Animal Biology, University of Geneva, 30 quai Ernest Ansermet, CH-1211 Genève 4, Switzerland and *Laboratory of Ocular Pharmacology and Physiology, University Eye Clinic, University of Basel, Mittlere Strasse 91, CH-4012 Basel, Switzerland.

In porcine coronary artery, bradykinin-induced endothelium-dependent vasodilatations are associated with simultaneous endothelium as well as endothelium-dependent smooth muscle cell hyperpolarizations. In contrast, in porcine ciliary artery bradykinin evokes endothelium-dependent relaxations, but no change in smooth muscle cell membrane potential.

This study addresses whether the lack of bradykinin-induced smooth muscle cell hyperpolarization is also associated with an absence of endothelial hyperpolarization in porcine ciliary artery.

With a microelectrode to impale cells in arterial strips, a 12 mV transient bradykinin-induced hyperpolarization was measured in endothelial cells. Bradykinin evoked no smooth muscle cell hyperpolarization deep in the media. Only occasionally, a slight 4 mV hyperpolarization could be recorded in some smooth muscle cells next to the endothelium. The endothelial intracellular injection (through the recording electrode) of the fluorescent tracers, lucifer yellow or ethidium bromide, showed the existence of a heterocellular dye-coupling between endothelial cells and smooth muscle cells.

These observations in porcine ciliary artery demonstrate that the lack of bradykinin-induced endothelium-dependent smooth muscle cell hyperpolarization is not due to an absence of endothelial cell hyperpolarization, but most likely of an insufficient electrotonic propagation space constant from endothelial cells to smooth muscle cell, despite the presence of a dye-coupling between these cells.

007

ENDOTHELIAL FUNCTION OF INTERNAL MAMMARY ARTERY. SIMILARITIES BETWEEN ADVANCED ATHEROSCLEROSIS AND HEART TRANSPLANTATION

P. Unger, V. Crasset, C.Giot, J-L. Vachiery, G.Berkenboom
Cardiology Department, Erasme Hospital, Brussels

To determine whether the endothelial function of internal mammary artery is influenced by the clinical conditions, the responses to increasing concentrations of acetylcholine (1, 10, 20 µg/min for 2.5 min each) were assessed in 6 control subjects (group A), 16 coronary patients (group B) matched with 16 heart graft recipients (for non ischemic cardiomyopathy, group C) and 12 coronary patients with advanced atherosclerosis (group D). Diameters were measured by quantitative angiography and the changes in % of base line were as follows:

	Control mm	Ach 1µg %	Ach 10µg %	Ach 20µg %
Group A	1.9±0.1	23±4	25±3	26±3
Group B	2.0±0.1	9±2**	17±1*	23±2
Group C	2.0±0.1	6±2***	9±2§***	12±2§***
Group D	2.0±0.1	3±1***	4±1§***	6±2§***

***P<0.001, **P<0.01, *P<0.05 vs group A; § P<0.01 vs group B. In some patients of group B, C and D (n = 6, 5, 7), Ach responses were reassessed after selective infusion of L-arginine; the maximal response to Ach was unchanged in group B but significantly increased in group C and D . Thus, some coronary patients, mainly with advanced atherosclerosis and transplant recipients exhibit an endothelial dysfunction of their internal mammary artery.

008

RAMIPRIL PREVENTS ENDOTHELIAL DYSFUNCTION INDUCED BY OXIDIZED LDL.

G. Berkenboom, I. Langer, A. El Ajani, Y. Carpentier, J. Fontaine.
Department Cardiology, Erasme Hospital, Brussels, Belgium

Oxidized LDL plays a key role in hypercholesterolemia-induced impairment of endothelium-derived NO-mediated responses. To assess whether long-term ACE inhibition may prevent this endothelial dysfunction, 4 groups of rats were treated in parallel; group 1 received ramipril 10 mg/kg/day p.o. for 6 weeks; group 2 received ramipril 10 mg/kg/day p.o. for 4 weeks and the last 2 weeks a cotreatment with ramipril plus HOE140 (a bradykinin B_2 antagonist 500 µg/kg/day, sub-cutaneous injections); group 3 received ramipril 1 mg/kg/day p.o. for 6 weeks; group 4 served as control. Rings of thoracic aorta from these groups were contracted by phenylephrine and relaxations to acetylcholine were determined in the absence and in the presence of human Cu^{2+}-oxidized LDL (300 µg/ml, 30 min preincubation). Oxidized LDL significantly attenuated these relaxations in groups 2 and 4 but not in groups 1 and 3. This toxic effect of oxLDL is directly related to the NO synthase pathway as L-arginine (0.3 mM) coincubated with oxLDL completely prevented the endothelial dysfunction in control group. Aortic cyclicGMP content, reflecting NO availability, was significantly increased in groups 1 and 3 but not in the 2 other groups. Thus, long-term ACE inhibition protects against the acute toxicity of oxLDL; the mechanism is bradykinin-dependent and seems to involve an upregulation of EDNO synthase pathway via B_2 kinin receptor.

009

EFFECTS OF INSULIN ON ARTERIOLAR DILATION AFTER NO SYNTHASE AND TYROSINE KINASE INHIBITION IN HAMSTER CHEEK POUCH MICROCIRCULATION

S. Bertuglia, A. Colantuoni
CNR Institute of Clinical Physiology, University of Pisa, 56100 Pisa, Italy.

A previous study on isolated skeletal muscle arterioles showed that dilation to insulin is endothelium dependent. We investigated if insulin effects on arteriolar tone might be related to tyrosine kinase cytoplasmic signalling. We determined the effects of insulin on arteriolar dilation in the cheek pouch arterioles on presence of NO synthase and tyrosine kinase inhibitors, N^G-monomethyl-L-arginine (L-NMMA) and genistein, respectively. Hamster cheek pouch microcirculation was visualized by a fluorescent microscopy technique. Arteriolar responses were evaluated after topical application of insulin and genistein on cheek pouch microcirculation, while L-NMMA was intravenously injected. Vessel diameters and arteriolar red blood cell velocity were measured by shearing monitor and dual window techniques, respectively. Insulin caused dilation of arterioles with diameter >40 and <20 µm by 16±4% and 30±5% of baseline values, respectively. After L-NMMA and insulin diameters increased by 12±3% and 10±2%, respectively. After genistein and insulin arterioles dilated by 13±4% and 24±4%. L-NMMA plus genistein abolished insulin induced vasodilation. In conclusion, dilation to insulin in cheek pouch arterioles might be mediated by a pathway involving NO and tyrosine kinase activation.

010

AUTOREGULATION OF THE CEREBRAL CIRCULATION: THE INTERPLAY OF PIAL ARTERY RESPONSES TO PRESSURE AND FLOW AND VARIATION IN WALL DISTENSIBILITY AND MEDIA THICKNESS

J.A. Bevan, N. Thorin-Trescases, T. Posena, A. Gentry, J. Dodge, C.L. Walters*, R.D. Bevan
Totman Laboratory for Cerebrovascular Research, College of Medicine, University of Vermont, Burlington VT 05405 USA and *Neurological Surgeons, P.C., Phoenix, AZ 85004 USA

In health, cerebral blood flow is effectively maintained despite changes in central artery pressure. Some of the structural and functional characteristics of human (1000-200 µm i.d) and rabbit (350-200 µm i.d.) pial arteries participating in this regulation have been studied in vitro using wire myograph and video perfusion systems. Human pial arteries were obtained during neurosurgical procedures. Wall distensibility, myogenicity and media thickness relative to lumen diameter increase as arteries get smaller. Both the magnitude and direction of the changes in tone in response to alterations in intraluminal flow vary with the level of pressure. The constrictor compared to the dilator component increases with intramural pressure elevation. Perivascular nerves have little influence on pial artery tone. It is presumably the interactions between these vascular wall features and the other factors involved in the regulation of the flow of blood to the brain that results in an arterial network that ensures an adequate brain blood flow under a wide variety of circumstances. This occurs with a minimum expenditure of energy. Autoregulation can be impaired after head injury, subarachnoid hemorrhage and stroke.

011

AN INDOMETHACIN-SENSITIVE MECHANISM MODIFIES INTRINSIC TONE OF PREMATURE AND NEWBORN HUMAN CEREBRAL ARTERIES

R.D. Bevan, E. Vijayakumaran, A. Gentry, T. Posena, T. Wellman, J.A. Bevan
Totman Laboratory for Cerebrovascular Research, College of Medicine, University of Vermont, Burlington VT 05405

The adult cerebral circulation autoregulates, and although the human infant brain circulation is not passive pressure regulated the effectiveness of this control and its basis is not known. Segments of basilar and middle cerebral arteries of 8 newborns (23 weeks gestation to term) were examined. Pressure perfused segments spontaneously developed tone, on average 40% of the maximum possible, and comparable to human adult pial arteries of similar size (300-1000 µm o.d.). Indomethacin (10^{-5} M) increased the tone. This effect was studied on isometrically mounted segments in myographs where indomethacin was found to either initiate tone or potentiate existing tone. In 7 of 8 infants tone was increased by 31.9 ± 8.3%. Indomethacin also potentiated responses to the vasoconstrictors norepinephrine (NE) and UK14304. Following washout of the vasoconstrictors angiotensin II (10^{-8} M) and NE (10^{-6} M), indomethacin caused a pronounced, sustained increase in basal tone. At the ages studied tone was also reversed by acetylcholine (10^{-6} M), isopropylnorepinephrine (10^{-7} - 10^{-6} M), histamine (10^{-8} - $3x10^{-6}$ M), papaverine (10^{-6} M) and intralumenal flow. We conclude that intrinsic tone is a prominent feature of these cerebral arteries and this and agonist-induced tone are modified by an endogenous indomethacin-sensitive mechanism.

012

HOMOCYSTEINE AND ENDOTHELIN AS DETERMINANTS OF ARTERIAL STIFFNESS IN END-STAGE RENAL DISEASE.

J. Blacher, K. Demuth, M.O. Benoit, N. Moatti, G. London, M. Safar
Médecine 1, Hôpital Broussais, 96 rue Didot, 75014 Paris, France.

To assess the principal determinants of arterial stiffness, we measured aortic (carotid-femoral), brachial (carotid-radial) and lower limb (femoral-tibial) pulse wave velocity in 74 end-stage renal disease patients undergoing hemodialysis (mean age ± standard deviation : 51.6 ± 15.6). We determined arterial blood pressure by sphygmomanometry, aortic calcifications by echography, routine biochemical parameters, total plasma homocysteine and plasma endothelin. Multiple stepwise regression analysis was used to assess the correlations between pulse wave velocity and determinants of biochemical and arterial parameters.

In this population, aortic pulse wave velocity was positively and independently correlated with systolic blood pressure ($p<0.0001$), age ($p<0.0001$), the prevalence of aortic calcifications ($p=0.0004$) and the prevalence of diabete mellitus ($p=0.0043$). The only determinant of brachial pulse wave velocity was mean blood pressure ($p<0.0001$). Lower limb pulse wave velocity was positively and independently correlated with plasma total homocysteine ($p=0.0001$), age ($p=0.011$) and plasma endothelin ($p=0.017$). Pulse wave velocity on any vascular site was not independently correlated with tobacco use, cholesterol, triglyceride, fibrinogen, hemoglobin, body mass index, or heart rate.

In conclusion, the determinants of arterial stiffness are different whether aortic, brachial or lower limb vascular site is considered. This study suggests that increased homocysteine and endothelin concentrations in end-stage renal disease may be of pathophysiological significance in the process of lower limb vascular remodeling.

013

NOVEL STORE-OPERATED CATION CHANNELS MEDIATE AGONIST-INDUCED CALCIUM INFLUX AND CONTRACTION IN RABBIT AORTIC SMOOTH MUSCLE CELLS

V.M. Bolotina, R.M. Weisbrod, M. Gericke, Y. Hirakawa, and R.A. Cohen
Vascular Biology Unit, Boston Medical Center, Boston, MA 02118, USA

Store-operated calcium influx is well described in non-excitable cells, but its nature and physiological significance in smooth muscle cells (SMC) is still unclear. Here we describe novel small (3 pS) nonselective cation channels (permeable to Ca^{2+}) which are regulated by the state of filling of IP_3-sensitive Ca^{2+} stores. Using patch-clamp recording of single channels and whole-cell currents, as well as measurement of Ca^{2+} influx, intracellular Ca^{2+} concentration, and smooth muscle tension, we show that these channels, but not L-type Ca^{2+} channels, mediate agonist-induced inward current, calcium influx and contraction of rabbit aortic SMC. Single nonselective cation channels were activated in cell-attached patches following depletion of Ca^{2+} stores by either angiotensin II (AII) or thapsigargin (TG) even when the rise in intracellular Ca^{2+} was prevented by BAPTA. AII and TG activated similar inward nonselective cation current and caused Ca^{2+} influx and Ca^{2+}_i rise which were inhibited by SKF 96365 and nickel, but not by nifedipine. AII-induced Ca^{2+} influx was prevented by inhibition of Ca^{2+} release from IP_3-sensitive Ca^{2+} stores. Thus, agonist-induced Ca^{2+} influx and SMC contraction is mediated by small nonselective cation channels which are activated upon depletion of IP_3-sensitive Ca^{2+} stores. Recognition of the ion channels responsible for agonist-induced Ca^{2+} influx and their mechanism of regulation has allowed a new understanding of both contraction and relaxation of SMC.

014

CAROTID PRESSURE–DIAMETER RELATION DURING DRUG INDUCED CHANGES IN ARTERIAL PRESSURE

I. Bonyhay[+],G. Jokkel[+],K. Karlócai[+], R. Reneman^, M. Kollai[+]*
[+]Clinical Research Department and 2nd Institute of Physiology, Semmelweis Medical University, Budapest, Hungary and ^Department of Physiology, Cardiovascular Research Institute Maastricht, Maastricht University, Maastricht, The Netherlands

In a frequently used technique to measure baroreflex sensitivity, the regression line relating changes in R-R interval to drug induced changes in systolic pressure is determined. It is not known if vasoactive drugs influence baroreceptor firing by affecting carotid sinus smooth muscle or simply by stretching the sinus wall, through changes in pressure.

The diameter of the carotid artery and its change with the arterial pulse was measured with ultrasonography (Wall Track System, Pie Medical, The Netherlands) in six young healthy subjects. Blood pressure was measured by Finapres. Phenylephrine and nitroglycerin doses were injected iv. to raise and lower pressure by approximately 15-25 mmHg.

Carotid dimensions increased in all subjects during the phenylephrine induced rise and decreased during the nitroglycerin induced fall in pressure. Distensibility decreased and increased, respectively. Diastolic diameter changed more than systolic diameter; changes were significantly different from control by single factor ANOVA and the Scheffe post-hoc test within individuals. The pressure-diameter relation exhibited a non-parallel "shift" upwards and to the right during the pressor, and downwards and to the left during the depressor response. The systolic pressure-diameter relation appeared to be non-linear, with a steeper slope above than below baseline. This relation appeared to contribute significantly to the non-linearity in the R-R interval – systolic pressure relation.

015

ALTERED FLOW-INDUCED DILATATION IN RAT CAROTID ARTERY WITH REGENERATED ENDOTHELIUM

C.M. Boulanger, S. Belmadani, E. Mathieu, D. Henrion, B.I. Lévy.
INSERM Unit 141, Hôpital Lariboisière, F-75475 Paris.

The purpose of this study was to evaluate in vitro the response of perfused rat carotid arteries with regenerated endothelium to changes in flow. The endothelium of rat left carotid artery was denuded using a balloon catheter (size 2F, uninflated) and was allowed to regenerate in vivo.

Four weeks after endothelial abrasion, the left carotid arteries with control or regenerated endothelium were excised, placed in a bath, and perfused with a modified Krebs-Ringer solution containing 10 mM HEPES and 4% albumin (flow rate 0-2 ml/min) under pressure (100 mmHg); the diameter of the artery was measured with the means of an ultrasonic echo-tracking system (12 MHz).

Under no flow conditions, the basal diameters of arteries with control and regenerated endothelium were 1135±30 and 1184±25 µm, respectively (n=4-6; ns). During stimulation with phenylephrine (10^{-6}M; decreasing the diameter by 177±23 and 168±22 µm), intraluminal acetylcholine (10^{-5}M) increased the diameter by 76 and 75 µm above basal resting levels in control arteries and in arteries with regenerated endothelium, respectively (ns). The response to increase in flow was estimated for each flow rate, as the difference between control conditions and after maximal vasodilatation (KCN; 100 mg/L). Increasing the perfusion flow from 0 to 2 ml/min (operating in vivo flow) augmented the diameter by 61±8 and 25±9 µm in control arteries and in arteries with regenerated endothelium, respectively.

These data suggest that in rat carotid arteries with regenerated endothelium, the endothelial response to increase in flow is impaired while that to acetylcholine appears to be unaffected.

016

VASCULAR ENDOTHELIAL GROWTH FACTOR (VEGF) ENHANCES THE EXPRESSION OF THE NITRIC OXIDE SYNTHASE III IN CULTURED HUMAN ENDOTHELIAL CELLS

A. Bouloumié, V.B. Schini-Kerth, R. Busse
Center of Cardiovascular Physiology, University Clinic of Frankfurt, D-60590 Frankfurt am Main, Germany

Vascular endothelial growth factor (VEGF) is a potent mitogen for endothelial cells that stimulates endothelial chemotaxis, vascular permeability and angiogenesis. Since nitric oxide (NO) has been shown to modulate endothelial cell growth, the effect of VEGF on the expression of endothelial NO synthase (NOS) III was examined.

Experiments were performed using primary cultures of human umbilical vein endothelial cells (HUVEC). NOS III mRNA expression was assessed by RT-PCR, NOS III protein by Western blot analysis, and NOS III activity by the nitro-L-arginine-sensitive increase in cGMP.

The NOS III protein content decreased with the state of confluency. Treatment of subconfluent endothelial cells with $VEGF_{165}$ (100 ng/ml) for 48 h did not affect the level of NOS III protein whereas it elicited a 1.9±0.2-fold increase in confluent cells which was associated with a 2.2-fold increase in the basal production of cGMP. VEGF increased the level of NOS III mRNA within 2 h which thereafter remained elevated for at least the next 48 h. The stimulatory effect of VEGF was concentration-dependent and was inhibited by the tyrosine kinase inhibitor, genistein.

These results indicate that VEGF enhances the expression of NOS III in HUVEC. Whether this stimulatory tyrosine-kinase-dependent effect of VEGF is due to an enhanced transcriptional rate of the NOS III gene or stability of NOS III mRNA remains to be elucidated.

017

POSSIBLE ROLE OF BASAL NO RELEASE IN HINDLIMB VASCULAR HYPOREACTIVITY AFTER MYOCARDIAL INFARCTION IN RATS

D.L. Brouwers-Ceiler, H.J.M.G. Nelissen-Vrancken, J.G.R. De Mey, J.F.M. Smits
Dept. of Pharmacology, CARIM, Universiteit Maastricht, P.O. Box 616, Maastricht, the Netherlands.

This study was undertaken to examine vascular contractile function in the perfused rat hindlimb two weeks after myocardial infarction and to assess the modulatory role of the endothelium therein.

Wistar rats were subjected to sham surgery (n=9) or myocardial infarction (MI; n=4). L-NAME (25 mg/kg.day s.c.) was infused in sham (n=7) and MI (n=7) rats for 2-weeks. Hindlimb perfusion was performed and potassium responses (K^+) and maximal resistance (Rmax) were measured. In separate groups (n=6-7), plasma nitrate levels were determined.

Vasoconstrictor responses were decreased in MI vs. sham. L-NAME pre-treatment decreased K^+ (14.7±1.3 vs. 21.9±0.9 mmHg.min/ml; mean±SEM) and Rmax (17.5±1.7 vs. 27.7±1.6 mmHg.min/ml) in sham rats, but had no effect in MI rats. Plasma nitrate was lower in MI than sham rats. L-NAME lowered plasma nitrate in sham rats to levels comparable to those in treated and untreated MI rats.

These observations are consistent with involvement of reduced basal NO-release in MI rats in vascular contractile dysfunction.

018

N-ARACHIDONYLETHANOLAMIDE (AEA) RELAXATION OF BOVINE CORONARY ARTERIES IS NOT MEDIATED BY THE CB1 CANNABINOID RECEPTOR.

W.B. Campbell, P.F. Pratt, W.S. Edgemond, C.J. Hillard
Department of Pharmacology and Toxicology, Medical College of Wisconsin, Milwaukee, WI, USA.

It has been reported that the endogenous cannabinoid, AEA, has the characteristics of an endothelial-derived hyperpolarizing factor in rat mesenteric artery [Randall MD et al. Biochem Biophys Res Comm 1996; 229: 114-120]. We have carried out studies to determine whether AEA affects coronary vascular tone.

The vasorelaxant effects of AEA were determined in isolated bovine coronary artery rings precontracted with U46619 (3 nM). AEA decreased isometric tension, producing a maximal relaxation of 51±9 % (n=6) at a concentration of 10 µM. Endothelial denuded coronary arteries were not significantly affected by AEA. The selective CB1 receptor antagonist, SR141716A (1 µM), failed to reduce the vasodilatory effects of AEA, suggesting that the CB1 receptor is not involved in this action of AEA.

Since AEA is rapidly converted to arachidonic acid in brain and liver by an amidohydrolase, we hypothesized that the vasodilatory effect of AEA results from its hydrolysis to arachidonic acid followed by conversion to vasodilatory eicosanoids. In support of this hypothesis, bovine coronary arteries incubated with [^{3}H]AEA hydrolyze 15% of added substrate; approximately 9% of the radiolabeled product was free arachidonic acid while the rest comigrated with prostaglandins. A similar result was obtained in cultured bovine endothelial cells. Neither whole vessels nor cultured endothelial cells preloaded with [^{3}H]arachidonic acid synthesized [^{3}H]AEA in response to A23187. These experiments suggest that AEA produces endothelium-dependent vasorelaxation as a result of its conversion to vasodilatory eicosanoids, such as PGI_2 or the epoxyeicosatrienoic acids. Supported by SSPHS grants DA09155 and HL-51055.

019

EPOXYEICOSATRIENOIC ACIDS ACTIVATE A K^+ CHANNEL IN SMALL BOVINE CORONARY ARTERIES THROUGH A GUANINE NUCLEOTIDE BINDING PROTEIN (G_S)

W.B. Campbell, P.L. Li
Medical College of Wisconsin, 8701 Watertown Plank Road, Milwaukee, WI 53226 USA

Epoxyeicosatrienoic acids (EETs) are endothelium-derived arachidonic acid metabolites of cytochrome P450. They dilate coronary arteries and hyperpolarize smooth muscles and are thought to represent endothelium-derived hyper-polarizing factors. The mechanisms of these smooth muscle actions remain unknown. This study examined the effects of EETs on large conductance, Ca^{++}-activated K^+ channels (maxi-K^+ channel) in small bovine coronary arteries. In cell-attached, patch clamp experiments, 11,12-EET (1-100 nM) produced 0.5-10 fold increase in the activity of maxi-K^+ channels. In inside-out excised membrane patch mode, 11,12-EET increased the activity of maxi-K^+ channel only in the presence of GTP (0.5 mM) or GTP and ATP (1 mM). This effect of 11,12-EET was blocked by addition of GDP-βS (100 μM). In outside-out patches, a specific anti-$G_{S}\alpha$ antibody (1:2000) completely blocked the 11,12-EET activation of maxi-K^+ channels. Anti-$G_{i\alpha}$ antibody, anti-Gβγ antibody and rabbit IgG were without effect. 11,12-EET failed to alter the calcium sensitivity of the channel. Cholera toxin (CT) causes ADP-ribosylation of a 52-kDa protein in homogenates of small bovine coronary arteries. This 52-kDa protein corresponded to G_S on western blot. Pretreatment with 11,12-EET decreased CT-induced ADP-ribosylation of G_S suggesting that 11,12-EET may ADP-ribosylate and activate G_S. CT, like 11,12-EET, increases the activity of maxi-K^+ channels. We conclude that 11,12-EET activates maxi-K^+ channel by a G_S protein-mediated mechanism. (Supported by HL-51055).

020

OUABAIN (OUA) ATTENUATES EPOXYEICOSATRIENOIC ACID (EET)-INDUCED RELAXATION AND HYPERPOLARIZATION OF BOVINE CORONARY ARTERIES

W.B. Campbell , P. Pratt, P.L. Li, and J. Kurian
Medical College of Wisconsin, 8701 Watertown Plank Road, Milwaukee, WI 53226 USA

Endothelium-derived hyperpolarizing factor (EDHF) has been identified as a soluble factor released by the endothelium to regulate vascular tone. Among the properties which separate EDHF from nitric oxide is the ability of OUA to block agonist-induced hyperpolarization and relaxation. Several studies indicate that the EETs, cytochrome P_{450} metabolites of arachidonic acid, represent EDHFs. They are synthesized by endothelial cells and relax and hyperpolarize vascular smooth muscle. To support this hypothesis, we have examined the effects of OUA on the electrical and mechanical effects of the EETs in bovine coronary arteries. These arteries relaxed in a concentration-dependent manner to 14,15-EET (EC_{50} = 600 nM), sodium nitroprusside (SNP) (EC_{50} = 200 nM), and bimakalim (BMK) (EC_{50} = 100 nM). OUA (10 and 30 μM) increased basal tone and blocked the relaxations to 14,15-EET but not to SNP or BMK. Resting membrane potential (E_m) of isolated smooth muscle cells (SMC) was -51±0.5 mV. OUA (30 μM) decreased E_m (-48.4±0.2 mV) whereas 11,12-EET (100 nM) increased E_m (-59.2±2.2 mV). OUA inhibited the 11,12-EET-induced change in Em (-50±0.8 mV). In patch clamp studies using the cell-attached mode, 14,15-EET significantly increased the open state probability (NP_o) of a calcium-activated potassium channel when compared to control cells (0.154±0.012 vs. 0.02±0.01). OUA alone did not change NP_o (0.01±0.01) but blocked the 14,15-EET-induced increase in NP_o. ^{3}H-OUA binds to SMCs (K_D=26±2 nM); however, EETs do not alter this binding. These results indicate that OUA inhibits EET-induced relaxation and hyperpolarization as has been reported for EDHF. These findings further indicate that EETs are EDHFs. (Supported by a grant from NIH, HL-51055).

021

PHENOTYPIC AND FUNCTIONAL CHARACTERIZATION OF REGENERATED ENDOTHELIAL CELLS AFTER BALLOON INJURY IN THE PIG

M. Castedo-Delrieu, M.P. Fournet-Bourguignon, J.P. Bidouard, I. Delescluse, S. Leonce, J.P. Vileine, P.M. Vanhoutte
Institut de Recherches Servier, 11 rue des Moulineaux, 92150 Suresnes, France

Primary cultures of endothelial cells from porcine coronary arteries with native or regenerated endothelium (4 weeks after balloon endothelium denudation) were compared. Using flow cytometry and microscopic methods, an increased heterogeneity in size with the presence of giant endothelial cells was observed in the regenerated population. Regenerated cells displayed a reduced ability to proliferate but did not show signs of apoptosis such as changes in DNA content, decrease of transmembrane mitochondrial potential or production of reactive oxygen species. Like native endothelial cells, regenerated cells could constitutively incorporate modified low density lipoproteins. However, the time course and dose-dependent uptake of fluorescent acetylated low density lipoproteins revealed an increased capacity of incorporation in regenerated cells in comparison with native cells, which suggests the overexpression of scavenger receptors. The same results were obtained with regenerated endothelial cells studied directly after harvesting from the coronary arteries.

These findings suggest that the regenerated endothelial cells display morphological and functional alterations that could be markers of the endothelial dysfunction observed in this model. Since modified lipoproteins impair endothelium-dependent relaxation, their abnormal uptake by regenerated endothelial cells could contribute to the altered vasomotor regulation described after balloon injury.

022

POTASSIUM CHANNELS AND ENDOTHELIUM-DEPENDENT HYPERPOLARIZATION OF THE GUINEA-PIG CAROTID ARTERY

T. Chataigneau, C. Corriu, M. Félétou, E. Canet, J. Duhault and P.M. Vanhoutte.
Institut de Recherches Servier, 92150 Suresnes, France.

The nature of the potassium channel(s) involved in the endothelium-dependent hyperpolarization induced by acetylcholine was investigated in the guinea-pig carotid artery by recording the transmembrane potential of vascular smooth muscle cells with intracellular microelectrodes. In the presence of inhibitors of nitric oxide synthase (L-NA) and cyclooxygenase (indomethacin), the hyperpolarization induced by acetylcholine was suppressed in the presence of elevated potassium in the superfusing saline solution. Glibenclamide, apamin, scillatoxin, charybdotoxin and iberiotoxin individually produced no or minor inhibition of the hyperpolarization. In the presence of the combination of charybdotoxin plus apamin or charybdotoxin plus scillatoxin, the effect of acetylcholine was abolished. The combination of iberiotoxin plus apamin was ineffective. Iloprost, and nitrovasodilators induced endothelium-independent hyperpolarizations which were blocked by glibenclamide but unaffected by charybdotoxin, apamin and the combination of the two toxins. In the presence of charybdotoxin plus apamin but in the absence of L-NA and indomethacin, acetylcholine induced an endothelium-dependent hyperpolarization. This hyperpolarization was still observed in presence of either L-NA or indomethacin. These findings indicate that, in the guinea-pig carotid artery, acetylcholine induced the simultaneous release of three hyperpolarizing factors (endothelium-derived hyperpolarizing factor: EDHF, NO and prostacyclin). The effects of NO and prostacyclin involve the opening of ATP-dependent potassium channels; EDHF the opening of an undetermined calcium-dependent potassium conductance.

023

NITRIC OXIDE UP-REGULATES A CALCIUM-ACTIVATED CHLORIDE CURRENT IN RAT AORTIC SMOOTH MUSCLE CELLS

T. Chataigneau, R. Tricoche, M. Joffre
Lab. Physiol. Régul. Cell., UMR 6558, 86022 Poitiers, France.

Nitric oxide (NO) exerts some of its effects through the activation of the soluble guanylate cyclase. Its putative influence on the chloride conductances in the vascular smooth muscle cells is still unknown.

We have characterized the calcium-activated chloride current ($I_{Cl,Ca}$) in the freshly dispersed rat aortic smooth muscle cells using the whole-cell configuration of the patch-clamp technique. This current was isolated with external and internal (pipette) high cesium chloride solutions to suppress the potassium currents.

$I_{Cl,Ca}$ is an outwardly rectifying current which does not inactivate and is significantly inhibited by DIDS, a chloride channel blocker. The threshold of intracellular free calcium concentration for the activation of the current is 100 nM. $I_{Cl,Ca}$ is activated by exogenous ATP. After pre-activation of the chloride channel by calcium, sodium nitroprusside, a nitrovasodilator, induces a biphasic and time-dependent increase of the amplitude of the chloride current, whatever the membrane potential. This potentiation is mimmicked by 8-bromo-cyclic GMP and inhibited by methylene blue. An inhibitor of the cyclic GMP-dependent protein kinase, H9, selectively prevents the second component of the potentiating effect of NO.

These results indicate that, in rat aortic smooth muscle cells, $I_{Cl,Ca}$ is up-regulated by the NO pathway, probably by two different mechanisms both involving cyclic GMP.

024

CANNABINOID CB1 RECEPTORS AND ENDOTHELIUM-DEPENDENT HYPERPOLARIZATION IN GUINEA-PIG CAROTID, RAT MESENTERIC AND PORCINE CORONARY ARTERIES.

T. Chataigneau, C. Thollon, J-P. Iliou, N. Villeneuve, M. Félétou, J-P. Vilaine, J. Duhault and P.M. Vanhoutte.
Institut de Recherches Servier, 92150 Suresnes, France.

Experiments were designed to determine whether or not the endothelium-dependent hyperpolarizations observed in the isolated guinea-pig carotid, rat mesenteric and porcine coronary arteries (in the presence of inhibitors of nitric oxide synthase and cyclooxygenase) can be attributed to the production of an endogeneous cannabinoid. Membrane potential was measured in the various tissues with intracellular microelectrodes. In the porcine coronary artery the hyperpolarization induced by bradykinin was unaffected by the synthetic cannabinoid antagonist, SR 141716 (1-3 µM), and the endogeneous cannabinoid receptor ligand, anandamide (30 µM), did not provoke hyperpolarization. In the rat mesenteric artery, the cannabinoid antagonist did not influence the endothelium-dependent hyperpolarization to acetylcholine. In the guinea-pig carotid artery, SR 141716 inhibited the response to acetylcholine but induced by itself a significant hyperpolarization of the smooth muscle cells. In these last two tissues, anandamide induced hyperpolarizations which were not affected by SR 141716 (1 µM). This hyperpolarizing response was not reproducible while acetylcholine was still able to hyperpolarize the tissue. The acetylcholine-induced hyperpolarization was unaffected by glibenclamide but abolished by the combination of apamin and charybdotoxin. Conversely, anandamide-induced hyperpolarization was significantly inhibited by glibenclamide but potentiated by the combination of the two toxins. These results indicate that anandamide (or an endogeneous cannabinoid) is unlikely to mediate endothelium-dependent hyperpolarization to acetylcholine.

025

IN VIVO EXPRESSION OF RECOMBINANT ENDOTHELIAL NITRIC OXIDE SYNTHASE GENE IN CEREBRAL ARTERIES

A.F.Y. Chen, L.A. Smith, M. Tsutsui, T.B. Crotty, T. O'Brien, Z.S. Katusic
Mayo Clinic, Rochester, Minnesota 55905, USA

The purpose of the present study was to determine whether the recombinant endothelial nitric oxide synthase (eNOS) gene can be transferred and functionally expressed in cerebral arteries in vivo. Replication-incompetent adenoviral vectors encoding a β-galactosidase reporter gene (AdCMVLacZ) or an eNOS gene (AdCMVNOS) were injected into canine cerebrospinal fluid (CSF) intracisternally (final viral titer in CSF 10^9 pfu/ml). After 24 and 72 hours, transgene expressions were evaluated. X-gal and eNOS stainings revealed adventitial transgene expression in major cerebral arteries. Electron microscopy immunogold labeling indicated that recombinant eNOS protein was mainly expressed in adventitial fibroblasts. Bradykinin-induced relaxations (10^{-10}-10^{-6}M) were significantly enhanced in AdCMVNOS-transduced vessels, either with or without endothelium ($n=5$, $p<0.05$). In AdCMVNOS arteries basal production of cGMP was significantly augmented, and the augmentation was abolished in the absence of calcium and significantly reduced by a nitric oxide synthase inhibitor L-NMMA. Contractions to uridine 5'-triphosphate (10^{-7}-3×10^{-5}M) or cGMP production were not significantly changed in AdCMVLacZ reporter gene-transducer arteries when compared with those of non-transduced control vessels. The present study represents the first successful in vivo eNOS gene transfer in cerebral arteries. This approach may help in development of gene therapy for cerebrovascular disease.

026

SOME CHARACTERISTICS OF EDHF-INDUCED RELAXATION AND HYPERPOLARIZATION IN THE RAT MESENTERIC ARTERY

D.W. Cheung, G. Chen. E, Burnette
University of Ottawa Heart Institute, 40 Ruskin St., Ottawa K1Y 4E9, Canada

The effects of EDHF released by acetylcholine (ACh) on membrane potential and relaxation were studied in noradrenaline-contracted rat mesenteric arteries pretreated with N^w-nitro-L-arginine (30 µM). When compared to NO, EDHF is more effective in eliciting hyperpolarization but less effective in inducing relaxation. NO (> 3 µM) elicited complete relaxation and a maximum hyperpolarization of about 7 mV. In contrast, ACh (0.5 µM) caused only a 50% relaxation with a 12 mV hyperpolarization. There were no increases in the maximum hyperpolarization or relaxation when ACh and NO was added simultaneously. When the arteries were maximally relaxed by NO (>3 µM), addition of ACh further increased the hyperpolarization.

EDHF release from mesenteric arteries could be detected in freshly isolated single cells from the rat tail artery. Using perforated-patch recording technique, membrane potential change was recorded from these detector cells. Direct application of ACh caused only depolarization and contraction of the detector cells. When perfused through the mesenteric arteries, ACh caused hyperpolarizations up to 12 mV and no significant contraction was elicited in the detector cells. The hyperpolarization response persisted in the presence of N^w-nitro-L-arginine. These studies indicate that NO differs significantly from EDHF in the hyperpolarization and relaxation responses. The bioassay studies indicate that EDHF is a transferrable factor.

027

TRANSDERMAL NICOTINE AND CORONARY ARTERIES

W. D. Clouse, R. D. Hurt, H. V. Schaff and V. M. Miller
Departments of Surgery and Physiology and Biophysics, Nicotine Research Center, Mayo Clinic and Foundation, Rochester, MN, USA.

Experiments were designed to determine effects of transdermal nicotine on endothelium-dependent responses of coronary arteries. Transdermal nicotine patches (either 11 or 44 mg/day, low and high dose, respectively) were applied daily to the shaved necks of male mongrel dogs. Untreated dogs were studied as controls. After five weeks of treatment, serum-nicotine averaged 5.1ng/ml and 16.8 ng/ml six hours after placement of patches in low and high-dose groups, respectively. Nicotine was detectable (11.0 ng/ml) only in serum from dogs treated with high-dose patches 24 hours after placement of the patches. Left circumflex coronary arteries were removed and suspended in organ chambers for the measurement of isometric force. In the presence of indomethacin (10^{-5} M), contractions to 60mM KCl were significantly greater in arteries from dogs treated with low- compared to high-dose nicotine patches. Endothelium-dependent relaxations to acetylcholine and adenosine diphosphate in arteries from dogs with low-dose patches were shifted to the right of those from control dogs and dogs treated with high-dose patches. Response curves to UK14304 and the calcium ionophore A23187 were similar among groups. These results indicate that transdermal nicotine causes time and concentration-dependent increases in serum levels of nicotine. Further, five week treatment with transdermal nicotine at doses used in humans and producing serum concentrations comparable to those in humans selectively affects receptor-coupled, endothelium-dependent relaxations in canine coronary arteries. These alterations may be associated with changes in depolarization of the smooth muscle.

028

NOVEL MECHANISM OF NITRIC OXIDE-INDUCED RELAXATION: ACCELERATED REFILLING OF INTRACELLULAR CALCIUM STORES AND DECREASED STORE-OPERATED CALCIUM INFLUX

R.A. Cohen, R.M.Weisbrod, M. Gericke and V.M. Bolotina
Vascular Biology Unit, Boston Medical Center, Boston, MA 02118, USA

Nitric oxide (NO) causes relaxation primarily by reducing intracellular free calcium (Ca^{2+}_i). We have described smooth muscle cation channels which mediate Ca^{2+} influx depending on the filling state of Ca^{2+} stores. These channels can be activated by depleting sarcoplasmic reticulum Ca^{2+} stores (SR) either with contractile agonists or by inhibiting refilling of SR by Ca^{2+}-ATPase (SERCA) with thapsigargin (TG). NO may inhibit Ca^{2+} influx and accelerate mechanisms of Ca^{2+} disposition including SERCA, plasma membrane Ca^{2+}-ATPase (PMCA), and the Na^+/Ca^{2+}-exchanger (N/C). Fura-2 was used to measure Ca^{2+}_i and Ca^{2+} influx through cation channels (as estimated by Mn^{2+} quenching) to examine the role of these mechanisms in the NO-induced decrease in Ca^{2+}_i in rabbit aortic smooth muscle cells. When Ca^{2+}_i was increased by angiotensin II (AII), NO accelerated the drop in Ca^{2+}_i caused by removing extracellular Ca^{2+}, implicating an activation of Ca^{2+} disposition mechanisms. Eliminating extracellular Na^+ and/or blocking PMCA with high Mg^{2+} and pH had no effect, excluding a role for N/C or PMCA. NO failed to decrease Ca^{2+}_i or Mn^{2+} influx increased by TG directly implicating SERCA. Also, the inhibition by NO of AII-induced Mn^{2+} influx was entirely dependent on the presence of extracellular Ca^{2+} consistent with the requirement to refill the SR. This indicates that the drop in Ca^{2+}_i caused by NO is initiated by SERCA refilling of SR Ca^{2+} stores. The decrease in Ca^{2+}_i is maintained by inhibition of Ca^{2+} influx through store-operated cation channels.

029

BLOOD FLOW DISTRIBUTION DURING ARTERIAL VASOMOTION AND VASODILATION IN HAMSTER SKELETAL MUSCLE MICRO-CIRCULATION

A. Colantuoni, S. Bertuglia
CNR Institute of Clinical Physiology, University of Pisa, 56100 Pisa, Italy.

We investigated blood flow distribution in microvascular networks, characterized by arterial vasomotion, during dilation and constriction induced by acetylcholine (Ach) and NO inhibitor N^G-monomethyl-L-arginine (L-NMMA), repectively. The skin fold window preparation was observed by fluorescent microscopy technique in awake hamsters. We measured diameter (D), vasomotion frequency with autoregressive method (VF) and red blood cell velocity (V_{RBC}) in A2 and A3 arterioles (Strahler ordering). The values were A2 D: 7.1±0.3 μm; VF: 6.5±1.5 cpm; V_{RBC}: 1.2±0.3 mm/s and A3 D: 15.5±2.2 μm; VF: 5.2±1.2 cpm; V_{RBC}: 1.4±0.4 mm/s under control conditions. Capillary V_{RBC} was 0.11±0.04 mm/s. During dilation there was a transient decrease in VF followed by a further increase in D with low VF (A2 D:+55±5, +80±6%; VF:5.5±1.2, 1.8±0.9 cpm; V_{RBC}: 0.6±0.2, 1.8±0.1 mm/s; A3 D:24±5, 38±4%; VF:4.7±1.3, 2.1±0.3 cpm; V_{RBC}: 1.4±0.4, 2.2±0.2 mm/s. Capillary V_{RBC} was 0.20±0.02 mm/s during maximal vasodilation. During constriction A2 D:-20±4%; VF:7.9±1.3 cpm; V_{RBC}:1.6±0.6 mm/s; A3 D:-15±3%; VF:6.3±1.2 cpm; V_{RBC}:1.8±0.4 mm/s were observed. Capillary V_{RBC} was 0.25±0.05 mm/s. In conclusion, microvascular blood flow increased significantly during maximal vasodilation without vasomotion.

030

ENDOTHELIUM-DEPENDENT ACTIVATION AND INHIBITION OF K^+ CURRENTS IN RESPONSE TO ACETYLCHOLINE IN SUBMUCOSAL ARTERIOLES OF GUINEA-PIGS

H.A. Coleman, H.C. Parkington

Department of Physiology, Monash University, Clayton, 3168 Victoria, Australia.

The currents activated by endothelium-derived hyperpolarizing factor (EDHF) in the smooth muscle cells of submucosal arterioles were studied using single microelectrodes and a switching clamp. Voltage ramps or steps were applied to determine changes in membrane conductance. Tissues were perfused with L-NAME (5×10^{-5}M) and indomethacin (10^{-6}M) to block production of nitric oxide and prostacyclin (PG) and the endothelium was stimulated with acetylcholine (ACh, 10^{-6}M for 30s). ACh evoked an outward current which was associated with an increase in the membrane conductance to K^+. Following removal of ACh, a slow inward-directed current occurred that was associated with a decreased membrane conductance and the inhibited current had a reversal potential at the equilibrium potential for K^+. Following destruction of the endothelium, the ACh-induced responses no longer occurred.

ACh can release factor(s) from endothelial cells which result in the activation and inhibition of K^+ conductances in arteriole smooth muscle cells. These responses can explain the hyperpolarization and an after-depolarization which occur in many blood vessels following stimulation of the endothelium. The factor(s) responsible are unlikely to be NO or PG, but may be EDHF and/or another factor.

031

ENDOTHELIUM-DEPENDENT HYPERPOLARIZATIONS AFTER CHRONIC TREATMENT WITH NO-SYNTHASE INHIBITORS.

C. Corriu, M. Félétou, L. Puybasset*, A. Berdeaux*, P.M. Vanhoutte.
Inst. Recherches Servier, 92150 Suresnes, France. * Dpt. Pharmacologie, Faculté de Médecine Paris-Sud, 94276 Le Kremlin-Bicêtre, France.

Membrane potential and changes in tension were recorded from isolated canine coronary arteries and guinea-pig carotid arteries and aortas to study the effects of chronic *in vivo* NO-synthase inhibition on endothelium-dependent hyperpolarization. In control canine coronary artery, acetylcholine and bradykinin induced endothelium-dependent relaxations which were unaffected by acute *in vitro* exposure to indomethacin, but partially inhibited by L-nitro-arginine (L-NA) or by the combination of L-NA plus indomethacin. In coronary arteries taken from animals chronically treated *in vivo* with L-NA, the response to the two agonists were significantly inhibited when compared to controls. However, in these coronary arteries, acute *in vitro* exposure to indomethacin, and/or L-NA no longer influenced the effects of both agonists. In the guinea-pig isolated aorta, the relaxation to bradykinin was abolished by chronic *in vivo* treatment with L-nitro-arginine-methyl-ester (L-NAME). In the guinea-pig carotid artery, (in the presence of L-NA and indomethacin) the acetylcholine-induced hyperpolarization was not significantly affected by chronic L-NAME. In the canine coronary artery, the hyperpolarizing response to acetylcholine was enhanced by chronic *in vivo* treatment with L-NA while the hyperpolarization to bradykinin was partially but significantly inhibited. These findings suggest that endothelium-dependent hyperpolarizations are maintained during chronic NO-synthase inhibition. The proposed negative regulatory role of NO on endothelium-derived hyperpolaizing factor production and/or release is not observed consistently.

032

ENDOTHELIUM-INDEPENDENT CYCLIC GMP FORMATION IN CAROTID ARTERIES OF DIABETIC RATS

F.R.L. Crijns, B.H.R. Wolffenbuttel, D.S. van Ingen Schenau, H.A.J. Struijker Boudier* and J.G.R. De Mey*.
Depts. of Endocrinology and *Pharmacology, CARIM, University Maastricht, The Netherlands.

The development of vascular complications in diabetes mellitus is often associated with endothelial dysfunction. Previously, we showed that cyclic 3'-5'-guanosine monophosphate (cGMP) production was reduced in denuded carotid artery segments of diabetic rats, compared to denuded segments of control rats, during stimulation with the NO-donor sodium-nitroprusside (SNP, 10^{-6} M).The present study was performed to investigate this disturbed response in more detail.

Diabetes was induced in Wistar Rp rats by streptozotocin (70 mg/kg, D, n=8). Control rats (C, n=10) received vehicle only. After 3 months, carotid arteries were isolated, mechanically denuded of endothelium and divided into 6 segments. Segments were incubated for 10 min in Krebs-Henseleit buffer in the presence of 3-isobutyl-1-methylxanthine with addition of SNP or S-nitroso-N-acetyl-penicillamine (SNAP) in 3 concentrations (10^{-6}, 10^{-5} and 10^{-4}M) during the last 2 min. cGMP was determined by RIA. Diabetic arteries produced significantly lower cGMP levels (fmol/μg protein $\pm$ SEM) during stimulation with 10^{-5} M SNP (197±27 vs 357±39, p<0.01) and 10^{-6} M SNAP (113±19 vs 243 ±19, p<0.01), whereas the maximal response to higher concentrations SNP and SNAP were comparable to those in control arteries.

We conclude that the carotid artery smooth muscle of diabetic rats is less sensitive to exogenous NO.

033

FLUORESCENT LIGAND BINDING TO RECOMBINANT ALPHA $_{1a/d}$ ADRENOCEPTORS

C.J. Daly, J.F. Mackenzie & J.C. McGrath
Clinical Research Initiative, Division of Neuroscience & Biomedical Systems, University of Glasgow, Glasgow G12 8QQ.

A fluorescent quinazoline (QAPB), similar to prazosin, has previously been used to visualise α-adrenoceptors on blood vessels and single cells (McGrath J.C. et al., T.I.P.S. 1996; 17, 393-399). We have now assessed the affinity of QAPB in competition studies with [^{3}H] -prazosin and compared the specific binding of [^{3}H]-prazosin and QAPB at $\alpha_{1a/d}$- adrenoceptors. Using imaging techniques the binding of QAPB to diffuse and clustered receptors has been examined. Rat 1 fibroblasts stably expressing $\alpha_{1a/d}$-adrenoceptors were grown to confluence and either seeded on coverslips or harvested for membrane preparation. Non-specific binding was determined in the presence of 10μM phentolamine in both tritiated and fluorescence saturation binding experiments. For fluorescence binding a confocal laser scanning microscope collected images of live cells at one minute intervals during incubation with increasing concentrations of QAPB (0.4-10nM). Inhibition of ^{3}H-prazosin binding to $\alpha_{1a/d}$-membranes by unlabelled prazosin, QAPB and doxazosin resulted in Ki values of 1.04, 1.24 and 17.8nM, respectively. Scatchard analysis of the specific binding curve for ^{3}H-prazosin binding to $\alpha_{1a/d}$-membranes produced a K_D of 1.89nM. Scatchard analysis of the specific binding curve for QAPB binding to $\alpha_{1a/d}$-'live' cells produced a K_D of 3.9nM. Using image masks for areas of diffuse and clustered binding it was possible, in individual experiments, to construct non-linear regression (saturation) curves of total intensity for different regions. The low (diffuse) and high (clustered) intensities produced almost identical fluorescence half maximal values of 1.9 and 1.6nM, respectively. In conclusion, QAPB is a competitive fluorescent α-adrenoceptor antagonist which can be used to visualise binding sites in living cells (at nanomolar concentrations) and enables the study of diffuse and clustered receptors.

034

3D-DISTRIBUTION OF α-ADRENOCEPTORS IN BLOOD VESSEL LACK OF STAINING ON ENDOTHELIAL CELLS

C.J. Daly, S.A. De La Rue, D. Luo, J.C. McGrath
Clinical Research Initiative, Division of Neuroscience & Biomedical Systems, University of Glasgow, Glasgow G12 8QQ

Fluorescent ligands and antibodies are becoming more widely used in localisation studies to visualise receptors in single cells and tissue slices. Recently, a 'prazosin like' fluorescent quinazoline (QAPB) was used to visualise α-adrenoceptors on recombinant cell systems and native tissue (McGrath J.C. et al., T.I.P.S. 1996, 17, 393-399). We have now extended these studies by examining the 3D-distribution of QAPB in segments of the mouse isolated tail artery (MTA) and rat isolated mesenteric arteric (RMA). Male mice (C57 black; 25-30g) or rats (Wistar 250-300g) were killed by stunning followed by cervical dislocation. Isolated RMA (2-3 rd order branches) were incubated in Krebs with or without a non-fluorescence antagonist. MTA was immobilised in a heated solution of glycerine and gelatine. After cooling, MTA was cut into 50 μm ring segments then attached segments to coverslips using Cell-Tak tissue adhesive. Coverslips containing M.T. segments were mounted in a flow chamber filled with 500 μl HEPE buffer. A confocal laser scanning microscope generated optical sections and full 3D-volumes of RMA (slide mounted) and MTA (coverslip mounted) segments (40x oil immersion; NA 1.3). MetaMorph and Imaris software provided analysis of 2D slices and 3D iso-surface volumes, respectively. QAPB (0.1 μM) bound primarily to the smooth muscle cells of the RMA Binding was in the form of bright clusters (covering 1.83% of the sample and a lower level diffuse staining (covering 71.2%). In the presence of 10 μM phenoxybenzamine the total fluorescence was 30.8% of control. No binding was observed in the endothelium of RMA. Examination of the 3D-distribution of QAPB (10 nM) on MTA revealed binding in the media and in the region of the internal elastic lamina. No binding was observed on the luminal surface of the endothelium. In conclusion, we have no evidence for QAPB binding sites on endothelial cells of RMA or MTA but can demonstrate their localisation at the sub-cellular level on vascular smooth muscle.

035

BLOCKADE OF PROSTANOID INDUCED SMOOTH MUSCLE CONTRACTION BY SULFONYLUREAS IS HETEROGENEOUS

C. Delaey, J. Van de Voorde
Department of Physiology and Physiopathology, University of Gent, Pintelaan 185, 9000 Gent, Belgium

Sulfonylureas are widely used hypoglycemic drugs. They stimulate the release of insulin by blocking ATP-dependent potassium-channels. We found on the rat aorta that the sulfonylureas glibenclamide (10 µM), tolbutamide, gliclazide and tolazamide (all 1 mM) block contractions with prostaglandin $F_{2\alpha}$, prostaglandin E_2 and the thromboxane A_2 mimetic U-46619, but not contractions with norepinephrine, phenylephrine, serotonin, endothelin-1 or K^+ (120 mM). Contraction induced by activation of G-proteins with AlF_4^- was also inhibited. Glibenclamide also inhibits prostanoid-induced contractions on other rat arteries (carotid, femoral and renal interlobar arteries) and on bovine retinal and ciliary arteries, but not those on aorta and carotid artery from guinea-pigs and on human subcutaneous arteries.

All sulfonylureas also block the contraction induced by U-46619, but not that with carbachol, on rat intrapulmonary bronchioles. However, prostanoid-induced contractions of guinea-pig trachea and main bronchi are not influenced by glibenclamide.

It is concluded that sulfonylureas exert a specific inhibitory influence on prostanoid-induced contractions of different types of smooth muscle cells (vascular and pulmonary). This inhibitory influence is heterogeneous, probably species-linked and might be due to interference with regulatory G-proteins.

036

K^+ AND Ca^{2+} CURRENTS IN BRAIN CAPILLARY ENDOTHELIAL CELLS ARE AFFECTED BY METABOLIC STRESS.

M.A. Delpiano
Max-Planck-Institut für Molekulare Physiologie, Rheinlanddamm 201, 44139 Dortmund, Germany.

Rat brain capillary endothelial cells (BCEC) were studied in voltage-clamp experiments with the patch-clamp technique to see whether they contain O_2-sensitive channels. Outwardly rectifying currents elicited from a holding potential (Hp) of -60 mV activated at -30 mV. Their tail current-voltage relation (I-V) reversed at -70 mV and shifted to more positive potentials at high $[K^+]_o$ (50-130mM). They were inhibited by TEA^+ (0.5-5mM), 4-AP (1-5mM), charybdotoxin (1-30nM), as well as tolbutamide (0.5-1mM) and glibenclamide (10-200µM). When using NMDG instead of Na^+ and K^+ ions in bath and pipette solutions, inward Ca^{2+} currents elicited from a Hp of -80 mV activated around -50 mV and had a maximum amplitude of about 160 pA at -25 mV. They were not sensitive to dihydropyridine derivatives (Bay-9644 (3µM), PN200-110 (10µM), nifedipine (5µM)), but almost totally blocked by amiloride and Ni^{2+} (IC_{50}: 25 and 32 µM, respectively). Lowering bath PO_2 from 38 (control) to 2.6 kPa (hypoxia) reversibly increased K^+ currents and hyperpolarized cells. Ca^{2+} currents were not changed. Cyanide (1-5mM), however, increased K^+ and depressed Ca^{2+} currents. 2,4-dinitrophenol (20-600µM) mimicked the effect of cyanide. The hypoxia-induced increase in K^+ conductance was prevented by tolbutamide (1mM) but not by TEA^+ (1mM). It can be concluded that BCEC contain voltage-activated K^+ and Ca^{2+} channels. These channels could mediate the microcirculatory response to metabolic stress, because they are affected by hypoxia and metabolic inhibition. The tolbutamide prevention of the hypoxia-induced K^+ increase suggests that ATP may be the intracellular signal.

037

BLOOD PLATELETS AS TARGET AND SOURCE OF NITRIC OXIDE. RELAXATION TO CALCIUM HANDLING

M.A. Devynck, F. Lantoine, K.H. Le Quan Sang, M.G. Pernollet, A. Brunet, F. Bedioui*, J. Devynck*
Pharmacology, Necker Medical School, René Descartes University, 75015 Paris; *Electrochemistry, ENSCP, Pierre et Marie Curie University, 75005 Paris, France

Nitric oxide (NO) is a potent inhibitor of platelet aggregation and Ca^{2+} mobilization in response to stimulating agents. The availability of a specific microelectrode to quantify NO concentrations in the nanomolar range has made possible the study of its acute effects on platelet Ca^{2+} handling and the quantification of its production in platelets. We demonstrated that:

* NO is functionally coupled to the Ca^{2+} pumps of the dense tubular system, with an inhibitory effect above 10 nmol/L and a stimulation below this threshold;
* in the absence of Ca^{2+} influx, NO addition to fura-2 loaded platelets increases the cytosolic Ca^{2+} concentration of non-stimulated platelets and reduces the Ca^{2+} mobilization induced by thrombin, thromboxane A_2 or thapsigargin;
* NO production is stimulated by collagen or endothelin-3, with a maximal NO production of 5 10^{-19} mol/platelet, but neither by thrombin nor by ADP;
* NO production does not parallel cytosolic Ca^{2+} changes, although it is decreased in platelets suspended in low Ca^{2+} medium or when Ca^{2+} transients are attenuated by an intracellular Ca^{2+} buffer.

These results reveal a new pathway by which NO can directly regulate cell Ca^{2+} handling and indicate that platelets activated by collagen constitute a vascular source of NO.

038

EFFECT OF NITRIC OXIDE SYNTHASE INHIBITION ON RESPONSES TO NORADRENALINE IN DIFFERENT SIZED MESENTERIC RESISTANCE ARTERIES

W.R. Dunn & S.M. Gardiner
Department of Physiology & Pharmacology, Queen's Medical Centre, Nottingham, NG7 2UH, UK.

We have examined the effect of the nitric oxide (NO) synthase inhibitor N^G-nitro-L-arginine methyl ester (L-NAME) on responses to noradrenaline (NA) in different sized mesenteric resistance arteries isolated from Brattleboro rats. Three branching orders of mesenteric resistance arteries; 1st order (passive internal diameter (ID) at 90mmHg; 350±15 (n=5)), 2nd order (ID; 297±24 (n=5)), and 3rd order (ID; 245±20 (n=5)), were set up in a pressure myograph and responses were obtained to NA (with propranolol (1µM) and cocaine (10µM) present), until artery diameter was reduced to ~50% of its passive diameter. This protocol was repeated in the presence of L-NAME (100µM).

Table 1 -log [NA] (M) required to reduce diameter by 10%

	control	+ L-NAME	conc-ratio
1st order	7.38±0.16	8.33±0.13*	0.96±0.15
2nd order	7.97±0.25	8.40±0.21*	0.43±0.20
3rd order	8.24±0.09+	8.46±0.08*	0.22±0.02[a]

Under control conditions, there was an increase in sensitivity of responses to NA as resistance artery diameter decreased (Table 1, +p<0.05, 1st versus 3rd order, Student's unpaired t-test). L-NAME enhanced responses to NA in all three branching orders (*p<0.05, Student's paired t-test). This effect was greatest in larger resistance vessels compared to smaller arteries ([a]p<0.05, 1st versus 3rd order, Student's unpaired t-test) such that, in the presence of L-NAME, there was no difference in sensitivity of responses to NA between 1st, 2nd or 3rd order vessels. Thus, we conclude that basal release of NO has a greater inhibitory influence over vasoconstrictor responses in larger compared to smaller mesenteric resistance arteries.

039

ROLE OF K^+_{ATP} CHANNELS IN CORONARY AUTOREGULATION

E.O. Feigl, D.W. Stepp, K. Kroll
Dept. of Physiology, Univ. of Washington, Seattle, WA 98195, USA.

Autoregulation, which is the intrinsic capability of an organ to maintain a constant blood flow despite changes in arterial pressure, is of special importance in the coronary circulation, because autoregulation allows the myocardium distal to a coronary artery stenosis to survive.

Coronary autoregulation was examined in anesthetized closed-chest dogs before and after K^+_{ATP} channel blockade with glibenclamide (1 mg/kg, iv), which also inhibits adenosine coronary vasodilatation. Coronary artery pressure was lowered in steps while coronary blood flow, arterial and coronary venous adenosine, lactate, oxygen and carbon dioxide levels were measured. Myocardial interstitial adenosine concentration was estimated with an axially-distributed, multicompartment model of adenosine kinetics.

K^+_{ATP} channel blockade decreased initial coronary blood flow 19% without a change in myocardial oxygen consumption, but the constancy (autoregulation) of blood flow with decreasing coronary pressure was not altered by glibenclamide. Interstitial adenosine concentration did not change in the pressure range 100 to 70 mmHg before or after glibenclamide, but did increase at 50 mmHg, indicating incipient ischemia. Coronary venous P_{O_2} and P_{CO_2} were little changed during autoregulation before K^+_{ATP} channel blockade, but venous P_{CO_2} increased with decreased perfusion pressure after glibenclamide, indirectly suggesting that K^+_{ATP} channels may contribute to autoregulation.

In conclusion, neither K^+_{ATP} channels nor adenosine are necessary to maintain coronary flow in the autoregulatory range of coronary artery pressure from 100 to 70 mmHg.

040

ENDOTHELIUM-DEPENDENT HYPERPOLARIZATION OF THE GUINEA-PIG CAROTID ARTERY AND CYTOCHROME P450-MONO-OXYGENASE.

M. Félétou, C. Corriu, T. Chataigneau, E. Canet, J. Duhault and P.M. Vanhoutte.
Institut de Recherches Servier, 92150 Suresnes, France.

The purpose of the experiments was to determine whether or not the endothelium-dependent hyperpolarizations observed in the isolated carotid artery of the guinea-pig (in the presence of inhibitors of nitric oxide synthase and cyclooxygenase) can be attributed to an arachidonic acid metabolite produced by the cytochrome P450 mono-oxygenase pathway. Transmembrane potentials of vascular smooth muscle cells of isolated carotid arteries of the guinea-pig were recorded with intracellular microelectrodes. When compared to solvant, epoxyeicosatrienoic acids (5,6-, 8,9-, 11,12- and 14,15- EpETrE), up to 3µM, did not influence the membrane potential. The endothelium-dependent hyperpolarizations induced by acetylcholine were unaffected by proadifen, metyrapone, clotrimazole (100 µM), quinacrine, eicosatetraynoic acid (50 µM) and 17-octadecynoic acid (17-ODYA: 5 µM). 17-ODYA at 10 µM produced a significant hyperpolarization of the resting cell membrane and a partial but significant inhibition of the acetylcholine-induced hyperpolarization. Apamin did not modify the effects of 17-ODYA but in the presence of charybdotoxin or iberiotoxin, 17-ODYA no longer influenced the resting membrane potential or the acetylcholine induced-hyperpolarization. These results indicate that, in the guinea-pig carotid artery, the involvement of cytochrome P450 pathway in the endothelium-dependent hyperpolarization to acetylcholine is unlikely. Furthermore, the unspecific inhibition produced by 17-ODYA can probably be attributed to the opening of large conductance calcium-dependent potassium channels.

041

THE CALCIUM-INDEPENDENT ACTIVATION OF THE ENDOTHELIAL NO SYNTHASE (NOS III) IS ASSOCIATED WITH ITS DEPHOSPHORYLATION AND SUBSEQUENT REDISTRIBUTION

I. Fleming, B. Fisslthaler, R. Busse
Institut für Kardiovaskuläre Physiologie, Klinikum der J.W.Goethe-Universität, Theodor-Stern-Kai 7, 60590 Frankfurt am Main, Germany.

We previously reported that shear stress and the tyrosine phosphatase inhibitor-induced production of NO is associated with enhanced tyrosine phosphorylation of Triton X-100-insoluble proteins. In the present study we investigated the effects of the protein tyrosine phosphatase inhibitor, phenylarsine oxide (PAO) on endothelial NO production, the membrane association of the NOS III and its phosphorylation. In the isolated, perfused, phenylephrine-constricted rabbit carotid artery PAO (10 µM) induced an endothelium-dependent vasodilatation which was insensitive to the removal of extracellular Ca^{2+} and the calmodulin antagonist calmidazolium (10 µM), but was abrogated by the tyrosine kinase inhibitor erbstatin A. In porcine aortic endothelial cells immunoprecipitation followed by phosphoamino acid analysis revealed that NOS III is phosphorylated on tyrosine and serine residues under resting conditions. Two tyrosine and serine-phosphorylated proteins (~97 and 220 kDa) were co-precipitated with NOS III. PAO promoted the dephosphorylation of NOS III as well as its associated proteins and was associated with the redistribution of NOS III to the Triton-insoluble fraction. The latter effects were sensitive to the tyrosine kinase inhibitor erbstatin A. These observations suggest that NOS III exists as part of a multimolecular complex and that its Ca^{2+}-independent activation seems to be linked to dephosphorylation of the enzyme and its associated proteins as well as the redistribution of the NOS III complex to the Triton-insoluble fraction.

042

INTERACTION OF 17ß-OESTRADIOL WITH NORADRENALINE IN RAT AORTA: A GENDER STUDY.

C. Forster, A. Fong, Y. Le Tran
Departmemt of Pharmacology, University of Toronto, Toronto, M5S 1A8, Ontario, Canada.

Declining oestrogen levels in post-menopausal women are believed to account for a predisposition to coronary artery disease. Hence, hormone replacement therapy appears to be cardioprotective, the mechanism for this remains unclear. It has been suggested that oestrogens exert a direct effect on the vasculature by inducing an endothelium-dependent relaxation response. Accordingly, we studied the interaction of 17ß-oestradiol with noradrenaline in endothelium-intact and -denuded aortic rings from age-matched (180-230g) male (N=4) and female rats (N=4). After testing for endothelial integrity, concentration-effect curves were constructed to noradrenaline (10^{-9}-10^{-4}M) and then repeated in the presence of 17ß-oestradiol (10^{-10}M).

Noradrenaline produced bell-shaped concentration-effect curves, the magnitude was greater in endothelium-denuded preparations and there were no gender differences (male intact, 0.92±0.09g; male denuded, 1.5±0.1g; female intact, 0.8±0.2g; female denuded, 1.3±0.2g). 17ß-Oestradiol significantly reduced the noradrenaline maximum response in only female, endothelium-intact preparations (no oestradiol, 0.8±0.2g; oestradiol, 0.17±0.05g). In addition, oestradiol shifted all concentration-effect curves rightward. This was greater in females.

Therefore, the mechanism for this interaction involves, not only, an endothelium-dependent component (females) but also an endothelium-independent process, which although less marked, does occur in males. The significance of these data imply that oestradiol affects vascular function in a favourable way in females and, to a lesser extent, males.

043

CYCLIC GMP IN CANINE CIRCUMFLEX ARTERIES FOLLOWING HEART FAILURE.

C. Forster, G. Larosa
Departmemt of Pharmacology, University of Toronto, Toronto, M5S 1A8, Ontario, Canada.

In heart failure, coronary arteries exhibit increased endothelium-dependent relaxations to acetylcholine. The mechanism for this response may involve increased activation of nitric oxide synthase resulting in enhanced production of cyclic GMP. Accordingly, we measured cyclic GMP in endothelium-intact and denuded coronary arteries treated with either acetylcholine or N^{ω}-nitro-l-arginine at control and heart failure. Twenty male mongrel dogs were divided into 2 groups (non-paced;N=9 and paced [250bpm for 4 weeks] to end-stage heart failure;N=11). Animals were killed and cyclic nucleotides were measured ($pmol.ml^{-1}$) in endothelium-intact and denuded arteries in response to acetylcholine (10^{-5}M) and N^{ω}nitro-l-arginine (10^{-4}M).

Basal cyclic GMP was lower in endothelium-denuded preparations (non-paced intact and denuded, 6.3±2.9 and 1.8±0.9; paced intact and denuded, 13.2±4.4 and 0.4±0.1). Acetylcholine-stimulated cyclic GMP was also lower in denuded preparations (non-paced intact and denuded, 30.1±4.4 and 3.1±0.7; paced intact and denuded, 27.9±4.9 and 0.7±0.4). N^{ω}nitro-l-arginine caused a depletion in cyclic GMP levels in both endothelium-intact and denuded preparations, although the depletion was not as great in intact vessels at heart failure.

These data suggest that the mechanism for enhanced endothelium-dependent relaxations in heart failure is due to a composite of increased basal nitric oxide synthase and a N^{ω}nitro-l-arginine resistant component in endothelium-intact arteries.

044

ALTERATION OF NITRIC OXIDE PATHWAY IN REGENERATED ENDOTHELIAL CELLS 28 DAYS AFTER BALLOON INJURY OF PORCINE CORONARY ARTERIES.

M-P. Fournet-Bourguignon, J-P. Bidouard, D. Saboureau, I. Delescluse, PM Vanhoutte, and J-P. Vilaine.
Institut de Recherches Servier, 11 rue des Moulineaux 92150 Suresnes, France.

The endothelium-dependent relaxations induced by serotonin, α_2-adrenergic agonist, thrombin, adenosine diphosphate and bradykinin are impaired in porcine coronary arteries after balloon injury.

To elucidate the cellular mechanism underlying the dysfunction of the regenerated endothelium, the NO pathway was compared in primary culture of native and regenerated endothelial cells obtained from porcine coronary arteries, four weeks after endothelium denudation. The cGMP in endothelial cells, reflecting their NO production, was measured under basal conditions and during stimulation with bradykinin. Using high performance liquid chromatography and ^{14}C-arginine as substrate, the basal NO synthase was estimated by measuring the citrulline formed by endothelial cells membranes. The cyclic GMP productions, under basal conditions and after stimulation with bradykinin, were decreased by 46 % and 71 % respectively in regenerated endothelial cells in comparison with the native cells. The activity of NO synthase was decreased by 30% in regenerated endothelial cells.

These findings suggest that the impaired capacity of regenerated endothelial cells to produce NO, both under basal conditions and during stimulation, can be explained partly by a reduced activity of NO synthase.

045

VASORELAXANT EFFECTS OF PIRETANIDE AND FUROSEMIDE IN GUINEA-PIG MESENTERIC RESISTANCE ARTERIES

J.L. Freslon, C.Gozalbes.
Department of Pharmacology, Faculty of Pharmacy, University of Bordeaux II, 146 rue Léo Saignat, 33076 Bordeaux Cedex, France.

The aim of this study was to determine if piretanide and furosemide, two loop diuretics, were able to exert direct vasorelaxant effects in guinea-pig mesenteric resistance arteries, as previously shown for hydrochlorothiazide (Calder *et al.* Eur J Pharmacol 1992; 220: 19-26).

For this purpose, guinea-pig mesenteric resistance arteries were dissected from non-drug treated animals and mounted in two-wire isometric myograph. Basal tension was determined using a passive extension protocol (mean diameter at 0.9 L_{100} = 334 ± 10 µm from 10 animals). Vasorelaxant effects of diuretics were studied in preconstricted arteries following depolarization with K-PSS (124 mM) or incubation with noradrenaline (50 µM). In the latter case, the effects of incubation with two K^+ channels inhibitors: iberiotoxin (blocker of calcium-activated K^+ channels, 100 nM) and glibenclamide (blocker of ATP-sensitive K^+ channels, 100 µM) were studied.

Both loop diuretics were devoid of effects in K^+-depolarized arteries. In noradrenaline-preconstricted arteries, piretanide and furosemide respectively induced dose-dependent relaxations with EC_{50} = 8,2 ± 5,9 nM (n=9) and 22,5 ± 10,1 nM (n=7) and maximal effects which represented 93 ± 3 % and 93 ± 2 % of initial preconstriction. In these conditions, relaxations were completely inhibited in the presence of iberiotoxin but unaffected by an incubation with glibenclamide.

No vasorelaxant effects were observed in the same experimental conditions in rat mesenteric resistance arteries.

These results show that, as previously observed for hydrochlorothiazide in the same arteries of the same species, piretanide and furosemide are able to induce acute vasorelaxant effects, which appear to be mediated mainly through an activation of Ca-activated K^+ channels.

Experiments are in progress to determine the role of endothelium in these effects.

046

DETERMINATION OF COMPONENTS INVOLVED IN THE FLOW-INDUCED DILATION OF A RAT PERFUSED CORONARY ARTERY

J-L. Freslon, P. Véquaud
Department of Pharmacology, Faculty of Pharmacy, University of Bordeaux II, 146 rue Léo Saignat, 33076 Bordeaux cedex, France

The study was designed to determine the endothelial factors involved in the flow-induced dilation of a perfused rat coronary artery. For this purpose, segments of the right interventricular coronary were taken from 10-15 week-old male Wistar rats. Vessels were mounted in an arteriograph where internal diameter was continuously monitored while intraluminal pressure was controlled. We have studied the dilation induced by flow (0-800 µl/min) in preparations showing a spontaneous myogenic tone following an increase in intraluminal pressure (90 mm Hg). This dilator effect was measured in control conditions, after incubation with L-NAME (100 µM), with indomethacin (100 µM), with TEA (5 mM) and after mechanical destruction of the endothelium (-E). Dilation was expressed as percent of the fully-dilated artery diameter (DI-SNP), and wall shear-stress τ due to the forces exerted on the wall of vessels was expressed in dyn/cm^2.

Our results (see figure) show that the flow-induced dilation observed in this preparation appears to be dependent on both the synthesis and release of NO and on the involvement of K^+ channels. In contrast, they do not support a significant involvement of a prostanoid vasodilating substance in this phenomenon. When endothelium was removed, a dilation was still observed and the mechanism(s) involved in this endothelium-independent component remain(s) to be determined.

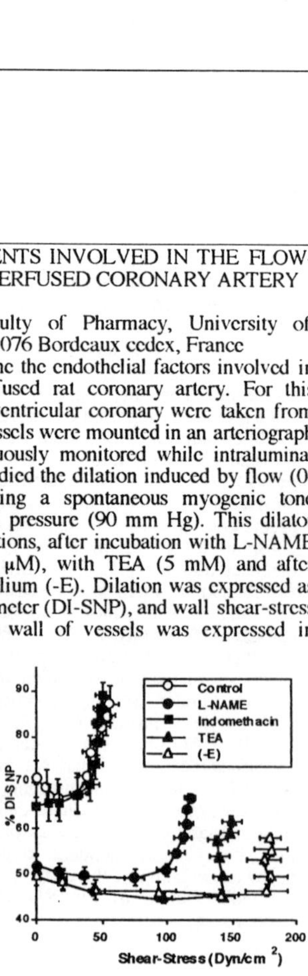

047

EPOXYEICOSATRIENOIC ACIDS ACTIVATE A HIGH CONDUCTANCE CALCIUM-DEPENDENT POTASSIUM CHANNEL ON CORONARY ARTERY ENDOTHELIAL CELLS.

M. Frieden, A. Baron and J.-L. Bény
Departement of Zoology and Animal Biology, University of Geneva, 30 quai E. Ansermet, 1211 Geneva 4, Switzerland.

Produced by the cytochrome P-450 mono-oxygenase in response to vasoactive blood mediators, epoxyeicosatrienoic acids (EETs) have been recently described as being endothelium-derived hyperpolarizing factors. The involvement of EETs during vasodilatation has been mostly studied with regards to their stimulatory effects on smooth muscle potassium channels (Campbell W.B. et al. Circ. Res. 1996; 78: 415-423). In the present study, we tested the effect of EETs on endothelial cells, focusing our experiments on the 285 pS calcium-dependent potassium channel, already described as being activated by bradykinin on pig coronary artery endothelial cells (Baron A. et al. J. Physiol. 1996; 493: 691-706). Potassium current was recorded from inside-out patches of cultured endothelial cells, EETs being applied on the cytosolic side of the membrane. In experimental conditions where the channel is partly activated (500 nM cytosolic calcium), 5,6- or 14,15-EET increased the channel open state probability by a factor of 2.5 ± 0.5 (n=5) and 4.0 ± 1.2 (n=4) respectively. This open state probability increase results from a mean open time and an opening number augmentation. Similar effects were also observed with 8,9- and 11,12-EET. These results show that in addition to their stimulatory effects on muscular potassium channels, EETs also activate calcium-dependent potassium channels on vascular endothelial cells, thus contributing to membrane hyperpolarization and cellular activation. Such autocrine effect of EETs must be taken into account, when implicating EETs as putative endothelium-derived hyperpolarizing factor.

048

VASCULOPROTECTIVE ROLE OF NITRIC OXIDE AT THE INFLAMMATORY CORONARY LESIONS IN PIGS IN VIVO

Y. Fukumoto, H. Shimokawa.
Research Institute of Angiocardiology and Cardiovascular Clinic, Kyushu University, Fukuoka 812-82, Japan.

We have recently developed a porcine model in which chronic, local treatment with interleukin-1β (IL-1β) causes coronary arteriosclerosis and vasospastic responses. This study was designed to examine how endothelial nitric oxide synthase (eNOS) and inducible nitric oxide synthase (iNOS) are altered in our model and whether these alterations are protective or injurious for the coronary artery. A segment of the porcine coronary artery was aseptically wrapped with either (1) IL-1β alone, (2) IL-1β+N$^{\omega}$-nitro-L-arginine methyl ester (L-NAME, an inhibitor of both eNOS and iNOS), or (3) IL-1β+aminoguanidine (AG, a selective inhibitor of iNOS). Immunostaining showed that iNOS was expressed only 1 day after the operation, while eNOS was well maintained. One day after the operation, coronary arteriography showed that L-arginine caused vasodilation only at the IL-1β-treated site but not at the IL-1β+L-NAME or IL-1β+AG-treated sites, while α2-agonist (UK 14304) caused vasodilation at the IL-1β-treated and IL-1β+AG-treated sites but not at the IL-1β+L-NAME-treated site, which indicated that L-NAME inhibited both eNOS and iNOS, while AG blocked iNOS alone. Two weeks after the operation, hyperconstriction to serotonin and mild intimal thickening were noted at the IL-1β-treated site, both of which were significantly enhanced at the site treated with IL-1β+L-NAME and with IL-1β + AG. These results indicate that NO produced by iNOS in response to IL-1β has an inhibitory effect on the proliferative/vasospastic changes of the coronary artery in vivo.

049

GENDER-RELATED DIFFERENCES IN PROTEIN TYROSINE KINASE MEDIATED COLD-INDUCED VASOCONSTRICTION

P.B. Furspan, R.R. Freedman
Dept. of Psychiatry, Wayne State University, Detroit, MI 48201 USA

Normally, in the absence of agonists, rings of rat tail artery do not contract when the temperature of the tissue bath is reduced from 37°C to 25°C. If, however, sodium orthovanadate (SOV, 100 µM), a relatively selective inhibitor of protein tyrosine phosphatase (PTP), is added to the bath 15 min prior to the temperature change, these rings will exhibit a small cold-induced vasoconstriction. This cold-induced vasoconstriction is more than twice as great in tail artery from females compared to those from males (13.4 + 1.53 % vs. 6.3 + 0.5% of 95 mM KCl response, $p < 0.01$, t-test, n=18). This cold-induced contraction was potentiated in vessels from both male and female rats by prior treatment with the inhibitor of nitric oxide synthesis, L-NAME (30 µM). When the plateau of the SOV-mediated cold-induced constriction was used as the baseline for a concentration-response curve to clonidine we observed that curves for both male and female rings were shifted to the left although to a greater extent for the rings from the males. Thus, SOV eliminated the gender-related difference in responsiveness to clonidine normally seen at 25°C. Tyrphostin 23 (50 µM), an inhibitor of protein tyrosine kinase (PTK), completely eliminated clonidine-evoked contraction in tail artery rings from both sexes and at both temperatures. These data support the hypothesis that PTK mediates cold-induced vasoconstriction in vascular smooth muscle. The greater responsiveness of tail artery from female rats compared to those from males (the result of greater baseline activity of PTK?) may be relevant to the pathophysiology of Raynaud's Disease (female to male ratio, 4:1). The clonidine results support the involvement of PTK in the mediation of alpha2-elicited contraction and may explain why alpha2-adrenoceptor-mediated contraction has been found to be potentiated in response to cooling in Raynaud's Disease. (Supported by NIH grant HL-30604)

050

REGIONAL VASODILATOR RESPONSES TO LIPOPOLYSACCHARIDE COMPARED TO TUMOUR NECROSIS FACTOR-α PLUS INTERLEUKIN-1β IN CONSCIOUS RATS

S.M. Gardiner, P.A. Kemp, J. Woolley* & T. Bennett
Department of Physiology and Pharmacology, University of Nottingham Medical School, Queen's Medical Centre, Nottingham NG7 2UH, U.K. and *Therapeutic Antibodies, Charterhouse Square, London, EC1M 6BQ, U.K.

Although there is evidence that lipopolysaccharide evokes cytokine release *in vivo*, it is not known if exogenous cytokines can mimic the haemodynamic effects of lipopolysaccharide. Therefore, in separate groups (n = 8) of conscious rats, chronically instrumented for monitoring renal, mesenteric and hindquarters haemodynamics, we assessed responses to lipopolysaccharide (2 mg kg^{-1} i.v.) or tumour necrosis factor-α (250 µg kg^{-1}) plus interleukin-1β (10 µg kg^{-1}).

The hypotensive effect of lipopolysaccharide (-25 ± 2.mm Hg at 1 h) was similar to that of the cytokines (-23 ± 2 mm Hg at 1 h). However, with lipopolysaccharide there was an increase in renal vascular conductance only ($+ 28 \pm 10\%$), whereas with the cytokines, renal, mesenteric and hindquarters vascular conductances were increased ($+53 \pm 7\%$, $+21 \pm 10$, and $+25 \pm 10\%$, respectively). Moreover, the renal and mesenteric vasodilator effects of the cytokines were apparent as early as 15 min from the onset of administration (vascular conductance: renal, $+32 \pm 8\%$; mesenteric, $+38 \pm 8\%$), although no hypotension was apparent at that stage. Fifteen min after lipopolysaccharide there was slight hypotension (-5 ± 2 mm Hg), but no regional vasodilatation.

The similar hypotensive effects of lipopolysaccharide and the exogenous cytokines at 1 h, in spite of the greater vasodilator effects of the latter, indicates that cardiac output was probably higher after administration of the cytokines. Thus, while lipopolysaccharide may stimulate the release of endogenous tumour necrosis factor -α and interleukin-1β, it probably causes, also, release of a cardiodepressant factor(s).

051

COMPARATIVE EFFECTS OF THE DUAL METALLOPEPTIDASE INHIBITOR, MDL 100,240 AND OF ENALAPRILAT ON REGIONAL AND ON CARDIAC HAEMODYNAMICS IN CONSCIOUS, HYPERTENSIVE, TRANSGENIC ((MREN-2) RATS

S.M. Gardiner, P.A. Kemp, F. Brunner* & T. Bennett
Department of Physiology and Pharmacology, University of Nottingham Medical School, Queen's Medical Centre, Nottingham NG7 2UH, U.K. and *Clinical Pharmacology, Hoechst Marion Roussel, Frankfurt am Main, Germany.

Heterozygous, male, hypertensive, transgenic ((mRen-2)27) rats were instrumented for the measurement of regional or cardiac haemodynamics and were given i.v. infusions of enalaprilat, or MDL 100,240 (both at 3 mg kg^{-1}, 3 mg kg^{-1} h^{-1}; n = 8 for regional and cardiac haemodynamics), for 32 h. Twenty four h after the onset of infusion of enalaprilat or MDL 100,240, the bradykinin (B_2)-receptor antagonist, HOE 140 (1 mg kg^{-1} i.v.) was given.

Over the first 8 h of infusion, both enalaprilat and MDL 100,240 had significant antihypertensive effects, accompanied by similar regional vasodilatations. However, the blood pressure lowering effect of MDL 100,240 (-54 ± 9 mm Hg) was greater than that of enalaprilat (-38 ± 4 mm Hg), because the former caused a significantly greater reduction in cardiac index. Between 8-24 h after the onset of infusion, there was a reduction in the hypotensive effect of enalaprilat, because cardiac index rose. In contrast, the antihypertensive effect of MDL 100,240 persisted, in spite of a recovery in cardiac index, because there was further vasodilatation, particularly in the mesenteric and hindquarters vascular beds. There were no apparent haemodynamic changes associated with the injection of HOE 140. These results are consistent with the antihypertensive effects of enalaprilat or MDL 100,240 in transgenic ((mRen-2)27) rats being due to suppression of angiotensin II production, rather than bradykinin degradation. The additional effects of MDL 100,240 are most simply accounted for by inhibition of the degradation of natriuretic peptides enhancing their effects on plasma volume, initially, and vascular tone, subsequently.

052

HYPOTENSIVE AND VASODILATOR RESPONSES TO HUMAN RECOMBINANT INTERLEUKIN-1β IN CONSCIOUS RATS

S.M. Gardiner, P.A. Kemp, J. Woolley* & T. Bennett
Department of Physiology and Pharmacology, University of Nottingham Medical School, Queen's Medical Centre, Nottingham NG7 2UH, U.K. and *Therapeutic Antibodies, Charterhouse Square, London, EC1M 6BQ, U.K.

Recent studies in conscious rats described pressor and tachycardic effects of interleukin-1β, with no signs of hypotension or vasodilatation, in spite of evidence that this cytokine activates vasodilator systems *in vitro*. Therefore, we have assessed regional haemodynamic responses to i.v. interleukin-1β at doses of 1, 10 or 100 μg kg^{-1}, infused over 45 min, and compared them to saline infusion, all in separate groups (n = 8 in each) of conscious, male, Long Evans rats (350-450 g), chronically instrumented with pulsed Doppler flow probes (renal, mesenteric and hindquarters) and intravascular catheters.

Relative to saline, interleukin-1β caused hypotension which was maximal at 1 h (-14 ± 2 mm Hg with 10 μg kg^{-1}), and accompanied by increases in renal and hindquarters vascular conductance (+41 ± 11% and +49 ± 18%, respectively; there was an earlier mesenteric vasodilatation (+42 ± 5% at 15 min). Blood pressure recovered subsequently (+4 ± 2 mm Hg at 4 h), in association with mesenteric and hindquarters vasoconstriction (mesenteric vascular conductance, -18 ± 3% at 3 h; hindquarters, -29 ± 4% at 4 h). Our results indicate that interleukin-1β has *in vivo* effects consistent with activation of vasodilator systems. However, its haemodynamic effects are complex, due to involvement of vasoconstrictor mechanisms also.

053

FEMALE OFFSPRING FROM UNDERNOURISHED WISTAR RATS HAVE NORMAL BLOOD PRESSURE BUT ALTERED VASCULAR REACTIVITY

R.TGerber[1], K.Holemans[2], F.A Van Assche[2] and L.Poston[1]
[1]Fetal Health Research Group, Departments of Obstetrics and Gynaecology, [1]St Thomas' Hospital, Lambeth Palace Road, London SE1 7EH and [2]Katholieke Universiteit Leuven, Herestraat 49, 3000 Leuven

It has been hypothesised that poor nutrition in utero may "programme" for cardiovascular disease in adulthood (Barker et Al. Lancet 1993; 341: 938-941). Female pregnant Wistar rats were subjected to a semi-starvation diet (50% normal intake) or to a normal diet. In 9 female offspring (100-120 days old) of 8 undernourished rats and 9 female offspring of 9 normal diet rats, blood pressure and heart rate were evaluated using chronically indwelling femoral catheters. Vascular function was assessed in the remainder of the offspring using a small vessel myograph. There was no difference in blood pressure in offspring from undernourished (181 ± 4 / 115 ± 4 mmHg, n=9) or normal diet rats (176 ± 3 / 125 ± 3 mmHg, n=9; ns) nor in the heart rate (479 ± 8 bts/min vs 460 ± 8). Acetylcholine and bradykinin induced relaxation were significantly impaired in the small mesenteric arteries of the offspring of the undernourished rats (max. relaxation to acetylcholine, 87.7 ± 2.65, vs control 95.51 ± 1.36, p<0.05; bradykinin max relaxation 18.1 ± 1.90 vs 26.24 ± 1.86 p<0.01, n=11 offspring). In contrast relaxation to sodium nitroprusside was enhanced (p<0.05 by summary scores). We conclude that undernourished in pregnant rats does not lead to elevation of blood pressure in the offspring. However subtle changes in vascular function may occur by which endothelial dysfunction is counteracted by an increase in sensitivity to nitric oxide.

054

SELECTIVE LARGE CORONARY ENDOTHELIAL DYSFUNCTION IN CONSCIOUS DOGS WITH CHRONIC PRESSURE OVERLOAD

B. Ghaleh, L. Hittinger, S-J. Kim, R.K. Kudej, M. Iwase, M. Uechi, A. Berdeaux, S. Bishop, S.F. Vatner.
Dept. of Med., Harvard Med. School, & Cardiovascular Research Inst., Allegheny Univ. of the Health Sciences, Pittsburgh, PA 15212, USA.

To examine endothelial coronary (C) control with chronic C pressure overload (CCPO) in the absence of systemic hypertension, we investigated large C arteries (C diameter) and C resistance vessels (blood flow velocity CBFv) to a 20-sec C artery occlusion, i.e., reactive hyperemia (RH), and to the administration of acetylcholine (ACH, 3 μg/kg, iv) in 6 conscious dogs with CCPO and 7 control dogs (CON). LV/body weight ratio was increased by 89% in CCPO. In CON, ACH increased CD (0.20±0.05 mm from 3.88±0.47 mm). This response was blunted (p<0.05) in CCPO (0.07±0.03 mm from 4.61±0.50 mm). Similarly, flow mediated increases in CD following RH were reduced (p<0.05) in CCPO, but nitroglycerin mediated large C dilation was preserved. In contrast ACH and RH induced similar increases in CBFv in CON and CCPO. Peak systolic CBFv was greater, p<0.01, in CCPO compared to CON (94±17 vs 35±7 cm/sec), due to systolic C hypertension (230 vs 130 mmHg). Histological analyses revealed multifocal intimal thickening with disruption of the internal elastic lamina in CCPO accompanied by mal-alignment of endothelial cells observed in large C arteries, sparing resistance vessels. Thus, in CCPO endothelial control is impaired for both flow-mediated and receptor mediated large C artery function, which could be accounted for by the major morphological changes, sparing the resistance vessels. The mechanism may involve chronically elevated systolic C perfusion pressure and CBFv.

055

EFFECT OF ACETYLCHOLINE ON RESPONSES EVOKED BY NORADRENALINE IN THE SUPERIOR MESENTERIC ARTERY OF THE RAT

P. Ghisdal and N. Morel .
Laboratoire de Pharmacologie, Université catholique de Louvain, UCL 5410, B 1200 Brussels, Belgium.

Acetylcholine induces an endothelium-dependent relaxation by the release of different factors (nitric oxide, endothelium-dependent hyperpolarizing factor and prostaglandin). In order to investigate the mechanisms involved in the relaxation of the superior mesenteric artery of Wistar Kyoto rat, we simultaneously measured membrane potential with intracellular microelectrode and tension changes induced by stimulation of the L-arginine/NO pathway on artery rings contracted by noradrenaline or by high KCl solution. Cytosolic calcium concentration was measured in fura-2 loaded artery rings.

In noradrenaline-stimulated preparation, the relaxation induced by acetylcholine was accompanied by a hyperpolarization of smooth muscle cells and a decrease in cytosolic calcium concentration.The nitric oxide synthase inhibitor, nitro-L-arginine, decreased but did not abolish these responses. In the presence of nitro-L-arginine, the nitric oxide donors SIN-1 and S-nitroso-N-acetyl-penicillamine relaxed the contraction evoked by noradrenaline, abolished the depolarization and lowered cytosolic calcium concentration to its basal value. The effect of SIN-1 was resistant to charybdotoxin, a blocker of Ca^{2+}-dependent K^+channels and to glibenclamide, a blocker of ATP-sensitive K^+channels. Acetylcholine as well as NO donors relaxed KCl-induced contraction without affecting membrane potential nor cytosolic calcium concentration.

These results indicate that nitric oxide could interact with an early step in the response to noradrenaline in the supérior mesenteric artery of the rat.

056

EFFECT OF LACIDIPINE ON ENDOTHELIUM-DEPENDENT RELAXATION AND ENDOTHELIN-1 EXPRESSION IN BASILAR ARTERY FROM STROKE-PRONE RATS

T. Godfraind, O. Feron, S. Salomone
Laboratoire de Pharmacologie, Université Catholique de Louvain, Avenue Hippocrate 54, UCL 5410, B-1200 Brussels, Belgium.

Lacidipine, a 1,4-dihydropyridine calcium antagonist, exerts a protective effect in salt-loaded stroke-prone rats, reducing the occurrence of cerebrovascular alterations and delaying their onset. It is known that endothelium-dependent relaxations are impaired in vessels from stroke-prone rats. In this study we examined if lacidipine-treatment (1 mg kg^{-1} day^{-1}) could improve endothelial function in these animals. Salt-loaded stroke-prone rats received either ordinary chow or lacidipine-containing chow for six weeks (from the 8th to the 14th week age). Basilar artery was mounted in a wire myograph and stimulated with serotonin (1 μM). Acetylcholine (3 μM) was added on the plateau of the contraction.

Among basilar arteries from control rats 42.3% relaxed to acetylcholine, whereas 70.7% of basilar arteries from lacidipine-treated rats relaxed to acetylcholine ($P<0.01$). The mean relaxation to acetylcholine was also higher in basilar arteries from lacidipine-treated rats (Control, 9.4±1.8, n=71; lacidipine-treated, 16.8±2.8, n=41; $P<0.05$). Expression of preproendothelin-1 mRNA, detected in basilar artery by reverse transcription-polymerase chain reaction, was reduced in lacidipine treated rats.

The protective role of lacidipine in stroke could be due to this action on endothelin-1 expression blunting both the endothelin-1 inhibition of NO synthesis and the endothelin-1-dependent increase of blood-brain barrier permeabilization.

057

CHANGES IN THE POTASSIUM CURRENTS OF RAT AORTIC SMOOTH MUSCLE CELLS DURING POSTNATAL DEVELOPMENT

J.P. Gomez and N. Morel
Laboratory of Pharmacology, Université Catholique de Louvain, UCL/54.10, 54 Avenue Hippocrate, B-1200 Bruxelles, Belgium.

Postnatal period is characterized by important changes in the cardiovascular system. However, relatively few studies have been performed concerning the changes in electrophysiological properties of smooth muscle cells during postnatal period. Since K^+ currents play a key role in controlling cell excitability, we have investigated the role of arterial K^+ channels in aorta from neonatal (1 day), young (28, 56 days) and adult (84 days) Wistar rats.

By the whole cell configuration of patch clamp technique, two components of K^+ currents were identified and characterized in isolated vascular cells from the same aortas: a small Ca^{2+}-insensitive delayed outward K^+ current, largely blocked by 4-aminopyridine and a larger Ca^{2+}-sensitive component, blocked by tetraethylammonium. The density of the first component remained unchanged at all ages studied, whereas the density of the second one was very low in 1 day-old rats and markedly increased between 28 and 56 days.

These results revealed that during postnatal period changes occur in thoracic aorta reactivity, in relation with the modifications observed in electrophysiological smooth muscle cells properties.

058

MECHANISMS OF ENDOTHELIN-INDUCED REGULATION OF ENDOTHELIAL FUNCTION.

M.A. Grafov, A.V. Lapshin, O.V. Stepanova, Yu.A. Romanov, N.A. Medvedeva, O.S. Medvedev.
Department of Human and Animal Physiology, Faculty of Biology, Moscow State University, Lenin Hills, Moscow, 119899 Russia.

Endothelin-1 at various concentrations differently modulates vascular endothelial function. In vitro it is demonstrated by changes in endothelium-dependent relaxation. We investigated mechanisms underlying endothelin-induced regulation of endothelial function.

Endothelium-dependent relaxation was tested in rings of isolated rat aorta 1 hour after 30-min vessel incubation with the peptde.

Rings incubated with endothelin-1 up to 0.1 nM displayed slight augmentation of maximal responses to acetylcholine via stimulated production of endogenous nitric oxide. The peptide at concentration 1 nM induced increase in EC_{50} value of endothelium-dependent relaxation. In contrast, 10 nM endothelin-1 potentiated effects of vasodilator through stretch-induced increase in smooth muscle sensitivity to NO. Endothelin-receptor antagonists attenuated vasoconstrictor action of the peptide and abolished endothelial stimulation. Moreover, vessels preincubated with antagonists and endothelin-1 (1 or 10 nM) were characterized by potent rightward shift of dose-response curve to vasodilator. So, high concentrations of the peptide produce endothelial impairment independently of known receptors. This effect was not due toxic damage of vascular endothelium as it was evaluated in culture. Endothelin-1 magnified ionic permeability of the lipid bilayer membrane. Since vasodilation is associated with cell hyperpolarization, this effect may mediate peptide-induced endothelial disfunction. Thus, endothelin-1 dose-dependently regulates endothelial function via different pathways.

059

ROLE OF ENDOGENOUS ENDOTHELIN-1 IN THE REGULATION OF VASCULAR REACTIVITY.

Grafov M.A., Gavrilova S.A., Volkov V.N., Medvedeva N.A.
Faculty of Biology, Moscow State University, Lenin Hills, 119899 Moscow, Russia (mgrafov@3.human.bio.msu.ru).

Administration of endothelin-1 affects not only blood vessels tone but also their responsiveness to other vasoactive substances. In the present study we investigated whether endogenous peptide influences on vascular effects of drugs.

Artificial decrease in the level of circulating endothelin-1 was induced by active immunisation of animals against the peptide. Adult rats were treated with either the peptide conjugated with hemocyanin or hemocyanin alone (control group). At the end of three months period of immunisation the responsiveness of conduit (aorta) and of resistant (caudal artery) vessels were tested in vitro.

The immunisation markedly reduced plasma level of endothelin-1 (1.9 fmol/ml vs 4.9 fmol/ml in control group). It was associated with elevation in mean arterial pressure and in heart rate (by 14% and 10%, respectively). In that group rings of isolated aorta displayed leftward shift of curve of endothelium-dependent relaxation. In contrast, experiments on perfused caudal artery of immunised rats evaluated 2-fold suppression of vessel reactivity to acetylcholine. In rats with decreased level of circulating endothelin-1 dilatatory responses to sodium nitroprusside were slightly reduced than those of control animals.

In conclusion, depletion of circulating endothelin-1 induced significant changes in haemodynamics associated with altered endothelium-dependent and independent vasodilation.

060

VASORELAXATION IN RESPONSE TO BRADYKININ IN HUMAN VEINS AND ARTERIES IN VITRO: EFFECT OF ACE INHIBITORS

C.A. Hamilton, M. McIntyre, R. Williams, G. Berg, J.L. Reid, A.F. Dominiczak, Departments of Medicine and Therapeutics and Cardiothoracic Surgery, Western Infirmary, Glasgow, G11 6NT, U.K.

The aim of the study was to examine relaxation to bradykinin in human arteries and veins. Internal thoracic artery (ITA), radial artery (RA) and saphenous vein (SV) were obtained from patients undergoing coronary artery bypass graft surgery. Vascular reactivity was examined in response to phenylephrine, carbachol (C) and bradykinin (B). Relaxation was re-examined in the presence of L-NAME (100-500μM), KCl 20 mM or perindoprilat (P -10^{-7} -10^{-5}M) to assess the contribution of nitric oxide and hyperpolarising factor to relaxation and the ability of ACE inhibitors to modify responses to B.

Arteries showed greater relaxation to C whereas relaxation to B was greater in veins. Maximum relaxation to C 58±7%, 92±9%, 38±6%: maximum relaxation to B 34±4%, 36±11%, 74±3% in ITA, RA and SV respectively. L-NAME and KCl attenuated responses to C and B suggesting that both nitric oxide and hyperpolarising factor could contribute to relaxation. Treatment with P, the active metabolite of the ACE inhibitor perindopril, improved relaxation to B in SV but not ITA. In SV P10^{-5}M decreased EC_{50} from 3.0±1.0 to 1.2±0.2nM (p=0.002, CI 2.177, 6.823) and increased E_{max} from 74±3% to 78±2% (p=0.004, CI 2.90, 9.89). P10^{-7}M decreased EC_{50} from 1.4±0.2 to 0.5±0.2 nM (p=0.002, CI 33.2, 93.0) but had no significant effect on E_{max}.

A greater understanding of the mechanisms of vasodilatation in veins and arteries may in the long-term lead to new strategies for treatment and prevention of atherosclerotic disease.

061

GENE TRANSFER TO ATHEROSCLEROTIC BLOOD VESSELS

D. Heistad, H. Ooboshi, M. Murray, M. Lang, B. Davidson, F. Faraci
Dept of Internal Medicine, Univ of Iowa College of Medicine, Iowa City, IA 52242 USA

We have made several recombinant replication-deficient adenoviral vectors to study vascular physiology and pathophysiology. We transduced aorta in vitro from normal and atherosclerotic rabbits and monkeys with adenovirus that expresses the reporter gene βgalactosidase. Transgene expression in endothelium was much greater in atherosclerotic than normal rabbits and monkeys. To examine mechanisms of augmented expression, lipid-loaded endothelial cells were examined in tissue culture. Transgene expression was greatly augmented in lipid-loaded cells when an adenovirus with a CMV, but not RSV, promoter was used. In lipid-loaded cells, there was increased activation of NFκB and CREB, which may enhance activity of the CMV, but not RSV, promoter. Inhibitors of protein kinase C or tyrosine kinase reduced DNA binding activity of NFκB and expression of βgalactosidase. Thus, it may be possible to selectively enhance transgene expression in atherosclerotic endothelium using the CMV promoter.

Carotid arteries from normal and atherosclerotic rabbits were transduced to alter function. Relaxation to acetylcholine (not nitroprusside) was augmented after transduction of eNOS in both normal and atherosclerotic arteries. Transduction of adventitia alone was sufficient to augment responses to A23187 in normal arteries. Relaxation to acetylcholine was augmented by transduction of CuZnSOD in normal, but not atherosclerotic, arteries. We have been unable to alter function by adenovirus-mediated transduction of extracellular SOD. In summary, it may be possible to selectively enhance transgene expression in atherosclerotic endothelium, with a CMV promoter, and to alter vascular function.

062

IS EDHF AN ENDOGENOUS CANNABINOID (ANANDAMIDE) ?

Holland, M., Plane, F.*, Garland, C.J.* & Boyle, J.P.
Cell Physiology, Leicester University, PO Box 138, Leicester LE1 9HN
* Pharmacology Dept., Bristol University, Bristol BS8 1TD

A recent study described arachidoylethanolamide (anandamide) as a putative endothelium-derived hyperpolarizing factor (EDHF) in the isolated, perfused rat mesenteric bed (Randell MD et Al. Biochim Biophys Res Comm 1997; 229: 114-120.). This study further reported that anandamide- and EDHF-mediated relaxations were inhibited by the cannabinoid CB1 receptor antagonist SR141716A. We find that in rat mesenteric 3rd order mesenteric arterial rings, pre-contracted with 2μM phenylephrine, anandamide causes relaxation (EC_{50}=316nM (limits 501-220nM, n=12). The relaxant potencies of EDHF (MCh 1-30μM or A23187 0.01-10μM, 5μM indomethacin, 200μM L-NAME) and anandamide were not modified by SR 141716A, indicating that neither agent was acting through CB1 receptors. When tested against tone induced by 80mM K^+ neither anandamide nor EDHF caused any relaxation. Therefore, anandamide-induced relaxation of mesenteric artery, like EDHF, may depend on inducing hyperpolarization of the smooth muscle cells. We tested the effects of a number of specific K^+ channel antagonists, in order to establish which, if any, K^+ channels were involved. Glibenclamide (5μM) or apamin (50nM) did not affect anandamide-induced relaxation. However, iberiotoxin (IbTX, 100nM) caused a significant shift in the relaxation curve and apamin in the presence of IbTX abolished any response to anandamide.

These results suggest that anandamide is activating Ca^{2+}-activated K^+ channels to induce hyperpolarisation and therefore may be an EDHF. However, this effect does not appear to involve CB1 receptors.

063

RELAXATION TO BETA-AGONISTS IN PULMONARY ARTERIES IS MEDIATED BY A NITRIC OXIDE-DEPENDENT PATHWAY

D. Hucks, R. M. Priest, J. P. T. Ward
Department of Allergy and Respiratory Medicine, UMDS St Thomas' Campus, London SE1 7EH, U.K.

It has been reported in several circulations that vasorelaxation to ß-agonists is partly endothelium dependent. We have studied the role of nitric oxide in ß-agonist-mediated vasorelaxation of pulmonary arteries of the rat. Large (~1mm i.d.) and small (~300μm) pulmonary arteries were mounted on a myograph and contracted with 50μM prostaglandin $F_{2\alpha}$. Concentration-response curves were obtained for isoprenaline and salbutamol, and following inhibition of nitric oxide synthesis with 100μM L-NMMA. At high concentrations isoprenaline caused an α-adrenoceptor-mediated contraction, and experiments were therefore performed in the presence of 10μM phentolamine. Results are shown as mean ± S.E.M.

L-NMMA substantially reduced the maximum relaxation to isoprenaline in large arteries (38±4%, n=6 to 5±1%, n=4, $p<0.05$), but was less effective in small arteries (49±5%, n=5, to 27±7%, n=5, $p<0.05$). In the presence of the $ß_2$ receptor antagonist ICI 118551 (0.1μM) L-NMMA effectively abolished relaxation to isoprenaline in both large and small arteries. This suggests $ß_1$ adrenoceptor mediated relaxation is entirely dependent on nitric oxide in these vessels. L-NMMA also reduced maximum relaxation to salbutamol in large arteries (35±7%, n=6, to 8±1%, n=4, $p<0.05$), but was again less effective in small arteries (51±8%, n=6, to 23±1%, n=5, $p<0.05$). The majority of ß adrenoceptor-mediated relaxation in prostglandin $F_{2\alpha}$ constricted pulmonary arteries may thus be dependent on nitric oxide, with the degree of dependence being greater in larger arteries. Supported by the British Heart Foundation.

064

MECHANISMS OF CEREBRAL ARTERIAL RELAXATIONS TO HYDROGEN PEROXIDE

Y. Iida, Z.S. Katusic.
Mayo Clinic, Rochester, Minnesota 55905, USA

The present study was designed to determine the mechanisms of cerebral arterial relaxations to hydrogen peroxide. Rings of canine middle cerebral arteries without endothelium were suspended for isometric tension recording. Production of adenosine 3',5' cyclic monophosphate (cAMP) was measured by radioimmunoassay. During contraction to uridine 5'-triphosphate (UTP; 10^{-5} mol/L), hydrogen peroxide (10^{-6} to 10^{-4} mol/L) caused concentration-dependent relaxations. Catalase (1200 U/ml) abolished the relaxations to hydrogen peroxide, whereas superoxide dismutase (SOD; 150 U/ml), and deferoxamine (10^{-4} mol/L) had no effect. The relaxations to hydrogen peroxide were abolished in arteries contracted by potassium chloride (20 mmol/L). A cyclooxygenase inhibitor, indomethacin (10^{-5} mol/L), significantly reduced relaxations to hydrogen peroxide. In the presence of calcium activated potassium channel inhibitor, charybdotoxin ($3x10^{-8}$ mol/L), a delayed rectifier potassium channel inhibitor, 4-aminopyridine (10^{-3} mol/L), and a nonselective potassium channel inhibitor, $BaCl_2$ (10^{-4} mol/L), were significantly reduced. An ATP-sensitive potassium channel inhibitor, glyburide ($5x10^{-6}$ mol/L) did not affect relaxations to hydrogen peroxide. Hydrogen peroxide produced concentration-dependent increase in levels of cAMP. Indomethacin inhibited the stimulatory effect of hydrogen peroxide on cAMP production. These results suggest that hydrogen peroxide causes relaxations of cerebral arteries by 1) activation of arachidonic acid metabolism via cyclooxygenase pathway with subsequent increase in cAMP levels, and 2) activation of potassium channels.

065

ENDOTHELIUM-DEPENDENT AND -INDEPENDENT MECHANISMS OF VASODILATION BY CORTICOTROPIN-RELEASING FACTOR IN PREGNANT RAT UTERINE ARTERY

V. Jain[1], Y.P. Vedernikov[1], G.R. Saade[1], K. Chwalisz[2], R.E. Garfield[1]
Department of Obstetrics and Gynecology, The University of Texas Medical Branch, Galveston, TX 77555-1062, USA,[1] and Research Laboratories of Schering AG, Berlin, Germany.[2]

Segments of the uterine artery (outer diameter 300-400 μm) from day 18 pregnant rats were mounted in a small vessel myograph in Kreb's solution, contracted with norepinephrine (10^{-6} M), and the relaxant responses to corticotropin-releasing factor (10^{-10} to 10^{-6} M) were studied. Results: Corticotropin-releasing factor relaxed the uterine artery in a concentration dependent manner. The relaxation of the uterine artery by corticotropin-releasing factor was abolished completely by α-helical corticotropin-releasing factor 9-41 (corticotropin-releasing factor receptor antagonist, 10^{-6} M), and partially by mechanical removal of the endothelium, Nω-nitro-L-arginine methyl ester (10^{-4} M), or 6-anilino-5,8-quinolinedione (guanylate cyclase inhibitor, 10^{-5} M). In deendothelized preparations, the relaxation could not be inhibited by 9-tetrahydro-2-furanyl-9H-purin-6-amine (adenylate cyclase inhibitor, $2x10^{-4}$ M), glibenclamide (10^{-5} M), or tetra butyl ammonium (10^{-3} M). Conclusions: Endothelium-dependent vasorelaxation by corticotropin-releasing factor is mediated by nitric oxide via activation of guanylate cyclase. However, neither the cyclic nucleotides (cyclic adenosine/guanosine monophosphate) nor the potassium channels are involved in the direct relaxant effect of corticotropin-releasing factor on the vascular smooth muscle.

066

RELAXATION KINETICS OF THE AORTA IN Nω-NITRO-L-ARGININE METHYL ESTER TREATED PREGNANT RATS

V. Jain[1], Y.P. Vedernikov[1], G.R. Saade[1], K. Chwalisz[2], R.E. Garfield[1]
Department of Obstetrics and Gynecology, The University of Texas Medical Branch, Galveston, TX 77555-1062, USA,[1] and Research Laboratories of Schering AG, Berlin, Germany.[2]

Timed pregnant rats (on day 15 of a 22 day gestation) were implanted with infusion pumps containing vehicle (controls) or Nω-nitro-L-arginine methyl ester (50 mg/day). Pumps were retained until term (group I), or removed on day 20 (group II). Rats were sacrificed at term. Aortic rings were mounted in organ chambers containing Kreb's solution for isometric tension recording. The rings were contracted with high-K^+ (60 mM), and allowed to relax in normal-K^+ (5 mM) Kreb's solution. Relaxation kinetics were quantified as the time for 50% and 80% relaxation. After washing and rest, the rings were contracted with phenylephrine (10^{-5} M) and responses to cumulative concentrations of methacholine (10^{-9} to 10^{-5}) were studied in the absence and presence of L-arginine (10^{-3} M). Results: Responses to methacholine were fully inhibited in group I, and partially in group II, and the inhibition in both groups was fully reversed by L-arginine. Relaxation was significantly prolonged in groups I and II. Mechanical removal of endothelium caused a prolongation of relaxation in the control group, and a further prolongation in group II, but not in group I. Preincubation of aortic rings from untreated controls with Nω-nitro-L-arginine methyl ester (in vitro, 10^{-4} M) did not prolong relaxation. Conclusion: Nω-nitro-L-arginine methyl ester may cause prolongation of vasorelaxation by endothelium-dependent mechanisms other than inhibition of nitric oxide.

067

ROLE OF LOW DENSITY LIPOPROTEIN ON ADENOSINE RECEPTOR MEDIATED CORONARY ARTERY RELAXATION.

S. Jamal Mustafa and W. Abebe. Department of Pharmacology, School of Medicine, East Carolina University, Greenville, NC 27858, USA.

The influence of low density lipoprotein (LDL) on relaxation of porcine coronary artery rings evoked by the adenosine analogs, 5'-N-ethylcarboxamidoadenosine (NECA) and 2-p(2-carboxyethyl)phenylamino-5'-N-ethylcarboxamidoadenosine (CGS-21680) was investigated. Preincubation of rings with native LDL (n-LDL 100 μg/ml and 200 μg/ml) for 4 hr in the absence and presence of copper sulfate (5 μM) selectively attenuated the endothelium-dependent relaxations produced by NECA and CGS-21680. LDL also inhibited the production of nitric oxide (NO) evoked by NECA and CGS-21680 in endothelium-intact rings. These effects of LDL were associated with enhanced oxidation of the lipoprotein. The inhibitory effects of LDL on both tissue relaxations and NO production as well as its oxidative modification were all prevented by high density lipoprotein (HDL, 100 μg/ml). In contrast, a relatively short period (20 min) of incubation with n-LDL produced no significant alterations of the relaxations and NO production elicited by NECA and CGS-21680. Under these conditions, no marked enhancement in oxidation of LDL was detected. These results suggest that prolonged incubation of coronary artery rings with n-LDL causes attenuation of endothelium-dependent vasorelaxation and NO generation induced by adenosine receptor stimulation and these effects are associated with oxidation of the lipoprotein. Such modulation may be important in hypercholesterolemia and in the development of atherosclerosis.

(Supported by NIH grant HL-27339)

068

ALTERATION OF REFLEX CONTROL OF THE CUTANEOUS CIRCULATION BY ORAL CONTRACEPTIVES

J.M. Johnson and N. Charkoudian
Univ. Texas Health Sci. Ctr. San Antonio TX 78284-7756, USA

While it is clear that the control of skin blood flow changes among the phases of the normal menstrual cycle, it is less clear whether the synthetic hormones in oral contraceptives cause a similar modification. Even less clear is whether any such modification involves the non-adrenergic active vasodilator system. To test whether active vasodilator function is modified by the active hormone phase of oral contraceptive use, in 7 young women whole body heat exposures were performed with water perfused suits during that phase and during the placebo phase. Skin blood flow was monitored by laser Doppler flowmetry at an untreated site and at a site iontophoretically pretreated with bretylium tosylate to block, presynaptically, adrenergic vasoconstrictor function. At this latter site, only active vasodilator function is intact. Heart rate and sweat rate were also monitored as thermoregulatory effectors. The internal temperature at which vasodilation began (threshold) was higher during the active hormone phase at untreated sites (37.09 ± 0.12°C vs. 36.83 ± 0.07°C; $p<0.01$) and at sites pretreated with bretylium (37.19°C vs. 36.88°C; $p< 0.01$). Similar shifts in threshold were seen for sweating (37.15 ±0.11 °C vs. 36.94 ± 0.11 °C; $p<0.01$). Heart rate at 37 °C in the active hormone phase averaged 81 ± 12 per minute and 96 ± 15 per minute during the placebo phase. The sensitivity of the relationship of these effectors to internal temperature was not affected by the phase. Hence, the synthetic sex steroids in oral contraceptives alter thermoregulatory control generally, including the reflex control of the cutaneous active vasodilator system.

069

INHIBITION OF PHOSPHODIESTERASE TYPE V RESTORES ENDOTHELIAL FUNCTION IN CHOLESTEROL-FED RABBITS

M. Kengatharan, M. Konneh, D.W. Laight, M.J. Carrier, E.E. Änggård
The William Harvey Research Institute, Charterhouse Square, London, EC1M 6BQ, England.

Hypercholesterolaemia impairs endothelium-, nitric oxide-dependent vasodilation. This is reflected by attenuated acetylcholine-mediated decreases in the relative height of the dicrotic notch, a marker of arterial compliance, measured non-invasively by photoplethysmography. We have studied the ability of the novel phosphodiesterase type V inhibitor, 4-[2-(2-hydroxyethoxy)ethylamino]-2-(1H-imidazol-1-yl)-6-methoxyquinazoline, (ONO-1505) (Laight et al. Brit J Pharmacol 1996; 119; 130P) to improve endothelial function in cholesterol-fed rabbits in vivo.

Male New Zealand white rabbits were fed either control or cholesterol (1%) diets for 10 weeks. After mild sedation, an infra-red photoplethysmographic probe was then secured on the ear for arterial pulse recordings.

Intravenous acetylcholine infusion (0.4-2μg/kg/min for 5 min) maximally reduced the relative height of the dicrotic notch by 33±8% (n=5) and 16±10% (n=6) in control and cholesterol-fed rabbits, respectively. The response to acetylcholine in the cholesterol-fed group was improved to 30±9% (n=6) 10 min after a bolus dose of ONO-1505 (10mg/kg), becoming similar to the control group response before ONO-1505. However, this response was still impaired relative to the potentiated control group response after ONO-1505 (46±6%, n=5).

The data suggests that macrovascular endothelial dysfunction in hypercholesterolaemia may at least be normalised, if not reversed, by augmenting the intracellular accumulation of cyclic guanosine monophosphate in response to agonist-stimulated nitric oxide.

This work was supported by ONO Pharmaceutical Limited, Japan.

070

cAMP HYDROLYSIS IS DIFFERENTLY REGULATED IN COBBLESTONE AND SPINDLE PHENOTYPES OF BOVINE AORTIC ENDOTHELIAL CELLS IN CULTURE

T. Keravis, N. Komas, C. Lugnier
CNRS URA 600, Universite Louis Pasteur de Strasbourg, 67401 Illkirch, France.

Phosphodiesterases hydrolyzing cAMP have been investigated in two morphologically distinct phenotypes of bovine aortic endothelial cells in culture, namely cobblestone and spindle cells, which represent respectively resting and angiogenic phenotypes encountered in vivo. The basal overall cAMP-phosphodiesterase activity of whole cell homogenate was 52% higher in spindle cells. The addition of cGMP induced a 60% increase of the overall cAMP-phosphodiesterase activity in homogenate of cobblestone cells, and this effect was due to stimulation of PDE2, whereas it induced a 30% decrease in homogenate of spindle cells. The absence of cGMP stimulatory effect in homogenate of spindle cells was not due to PDE2 itself, since cGMP was able to induce a 5 fold increase of cAMP activity of cytosolic PDE2 purified by anion exchange chromatography from spindle cells. The cAMP-phosphodiesterase activity of cytosolic fraction was due to four isozymes (PDE1, PDE2, PDE3, and PDE4) in spindle cells, whereas it was due to two isozymes (PDE2 and PDE4) in cobblestone cells. The cAMP activity of PDE3, which was essentially particulate in cobblestone cells, was also detected in cytosolic fraction of spindle cells, and the 7.5 kb PDE3A-mRNA transcript was six times more expressed in spindle cells. The analysis of PDE4-mRNA transcripts showed that various PDE4 isozymes were expressed in endothelial cells: PDE4B was more abundantly expressed, but PDE4A and PDE4D were also present. PDE4B and PDE4A transcripts were more expressed in cobblestone cells, whereas the 7.0 kb PDE4D transcript was more expressed in spindle cells. These results indicate a differential expression of phosphodiesterase isozymes in the two phenotypes, with a higher cAMP hydrolytic activity in spindle cells, associated with a decrease of intracellular cAMP, level of which is known to be associated with proliferation and angiogenesis.

071

PROINFLAMMATORY MEDIATORS IMPAIR THE SYNTHESIS OF ENDOTHELIUM-DERIVED HYPERPOLARIZING FACTOR (EDHF) IN ARTERIES THROUGH A cGMP-DEPENDENT MECHANISM

P. Kessler, R. Popp, R. Busse, V.B. Schini-Kerth
Center of Cardiovascular Physiology, University Clinic of Frankfurt, D-60590 Frankfurt am Main, Germany

In the present study we examined whether proinflammatory mediators which impair endothelium-dependent relaxations and stimulate inducible nitric oxide synthase expression, affect the synthesis of EDHF in arteries.

Rabbit carotid arteries were exposed to interleukin-1 ß for 7 h and porcine coronary arteries were incubated for 15 h with a combination of tumor necrosis factor α, interferon γ and lipopolysaccharide. The EDHF-dependent relaxation was assessed in the organ bath, and the release of EDHF by a bioassay system measuring the hyperpolarization of detector smooth muscle cells in the presence of nitro L-arginine and diclofenac.

Treatment with proinflammatory mediators significantly impaired endothelium-dependent relaxation to various agonists, an effect which was partially prevented by the inducible nitric oxide synthase inhibitor S-methylthiourea, and mimicked by the nitric oxide donor CAS 4609. Relaxations to cromakalim were not affected. The perfusates from bradykinin-stimulated coronary arteries hyperpolarized detector cells: control, 17.4 ± 0.8 mV, proinflammatory mediators-treated, 8.6 ± 1.0 mV, CAS 4609-treated, 7.9 ± 0.4 mV and 8-Br-cGMP-treated, 9.7 ± 0.9 mV.

The findings indicate that proinflammatory mediators impair the EDHF-dependent relaxation in arteries, in part, by inhibiting the synthesis of EDHF in endothelial cells via a cGMP-dependent mechanism.

072

ATTENUATION OF CORONARY VASODILATATION BY MYOCARDIAL CONTRACTURE AFTER PROLONGED COLD STORAGE

E. Kevelaitis, S. Kevelaitiene, N.C.B. Nyborg[1], Ph. Menasché[2]
Dept. of Human Physiology and Clinic of Cardiology, Medical Academy, 3000 Kaunas, Lithuania; [1] Dept. of Biology, The Royal Danish School of Pharmacy, 2100 Copenhagen, Denmark; [2] Dept. of Cardiovascular Surgery, Hôpital Lariboisiere, 75475 Paris Cedex 10, France

The objective of this study was to assess the effect of myocardial factors on the coronary vasodilatation of isolated hearts subjected to prolonged cold storage. Isolated buffer-perfused rat hearts were stored at +4°C for 10 hrs either in saline (group 1), in Celsior®(group 2), in Celsior with 2 mmol/L of L-arginine (group 3), or in Celsior with both 2 mmol/L of L-arginine and 30 mmol/L of 2,3-butanedione monoxime, an inhibitor of cross-bridge formation (group 4). After storage, left ventricular pressure-volume curves were constructed. 5-hydroxytryptamine and papaverine were used to test changes in endothelium-dependent and -independent coronary vasodilatation, respectively, and compared with those obtained during preischemic period. The direct effect of prolonged cold storage either in saline (group 5), or in Celsior solution (group 6) on endothelial and smooth muscle function of isolated coronary arteries was assessed on the isometric wire myograph.

After cold storage, postischemic myocardial contracture was ameliorated in group 4. Endothelium-independent vasodilatory response was preserved in group 4, whereas it was reduced in groups 1, 2 and 3. Endothelium-dependent vasodilatation was lost after storage and reperfusion in all isolated hearts. Endothelium-independent relaxation and the maximal contractile response did not change after storage in groups 5 and 6 of isolated coronary arteries. The basal tone was increased and endothelium-dependent relaxation to acetylcholine reduced in group 5, whereas it did change in group 6.

In conclusion, myocardial contracture can reduce coronary dilatory reserve

073

THE ANTIOXIDANT 2-(ALLYLTHIO)PYRAZINE PREVENTS THE LIPOPOLYSACCHARIDE-INDUCED ATTENUATION OF CONTRACTIONS TO PHENYLEPHRINE AND CAUSES ENDOTHELIUM-DEPENDENT RELAXATION IN THE RAT AORTA

Nak Doo Kim, Keon Wook Kang, Sang Geon Kim and V.B. Schini-Kerth
College of Pharmacy, Seoul National University, Seoul, Korea, College of Pharmacy, Duksung Women's University, Seoul, Korea and Zentrum der Physiologie, Klinikum der JWG-Universitat, Frankfurt, Germany

Septic shock is characterized by a severe hypotension which is due, in part, to the induction of nitric oxide synthase (iNOS) by lipopolysaccharide (LPS) in the blood vessel. The aim of the present study is to determine whether 2-(allylthio)pyrazine (2-AP), an antioxidant, affects the LPS-induced generation of nitric oxide in the vascular smooth muscle as well as the LPS-induced mortality in vivo. The effect of 2-AP on the generation of nitric oxide by endothelial cells was also studied. 2-AP prevented significant attenuation of contractions to phenylephrine and immunodetectable induction of iNOS in rat aortic rings without endothelium exposed to LPS for 6hr. In addition, 2-AP caused endothelium-dependent relaxations of rat aortic rings-contracted with phenylephrine that were inhibited by either methylene blue or nitro-L-arginine. For survival studies, mice received a bolus intravenous administration of LPS (55mg/kg), and the number of surviving mice were determined thereafter. Intraperitoneal administration of 2-AP increased, in a dose-dependent manner, the number of surviving LPS-treated mice, this effect was associated with a significant reduction of the serum nitrite and nitrate levels. These results indicate that 2-AP prevents the LPS-induced expression of iNOS in the vascular smooth muscle and stimulates the generation of nitric oxide in endothelial cells. These effects may contribute to explain the protective effect of 2-AP in LPS-induced septic shock.

074

DELAYED, ENHANCED NO MEDIATED CORONARY VASODILATION FOLLOWING BRIEF ISCHEMIA IN CONSCIOUS DOGS

S.-J.Kim, B.Ghaleh, R.K.Kudej, C.-H.Huang, T.H.Hintze, S.F.Vatner.
Dept. Of Med., Harvard Med. School, & Cardiovascular Research Inst., Allegheny University of the Health Sciences, Pittsburgh, PA 15212 USA

The goal of this study was to determine both the early and delayed effects of a brief coronary artery occlusion (CAO) on coronary endothelial function. 14 dogs were chronically instrumented to measure aortic and left ventricular pressures, wall thickness, and left circumflex coronary blood flow (CBF). Before CAO and during CAR, coronary vascular reactivity was investigated by 15 sec CAO and subsequent reactive hyperemia (RH) and selective intracoronary (i.c.) infusion of acetylcholine (ACh, 10 μg/min) and bradykinin (BK, 2.5 μg/min), and sodium nitroprusside (SNP, 40 μg/min). CBF responses to ACh and BK began to increase at 6 hours after CAR and reached a peak at 1-2 day CAR, and then subsided over the subsequent 4 days. At 1 day after CAR, enhanced CBF responses, compared to pre-CAO, were observed for ACh (66 ± 20 %) and BK (74 ± 24 %), and RH (24 ± 5 %), but not to SNP (-2 ± 10)($p<0.05$). Production of nitric oxide (NO) metabolites (nitrate and nitrite) measured as their coronary arteriovenous difference x CBF was increased at both baseline (153 ± 56 %) and during BK (220 ± 76 %) ($p<0.05$). Furthermore, i.c. pretreatment with NOS inhibitor prior to CAO and 1 day CAR, N^G-nitro-L-arginine (L-NA, 50 mg), prevented the delayed, enhanced endothelial function. Thus, in contrast to previous studies, these data indicate that brief ischemic episodes induce enhanced coronary endothelial function, which is delayed in onset and prolonged in duration which can be explained by an upregulation of coronary vascular NO.

075

ADVENTITIA DERIVED NITRIC OXIDE TRIGGERED BY LIPOPOLYSACCHARIDE IN RAT AORTA

A.L. Kleschyov, B. Muller, T. Keravis, J.C. Stoclet
Laboratoire de Pharmacologie et Physiopathologie Cellulaires,Université Louis Pasteur de Strasbourg, CNRS URA 600, 67401 Illkirch, France

It is well known that in blood vessels, bacterial lipopolysaccharide induces the L-arginine/NO/cyclic GMP pathway, leading to vasodilatation and hyporeactivity to catecholamines. In this situation, it is generally accepted that nitric oxide originates from smooth muscle cells themselves. In the present study, we wondered whether tunica adventitia, which contains fibroblasts and macrophages, could generate appreciable amounts of nitric oxide in response to the challenge with endotoxin.

In *in vitro* experiments, whole thoracic aortae were incubated in the presence of lipopolysaccharide (10μg/ml) for 20h. In *ex vivo* experiments lipopolysaccharide (40mg/kg; i.p.) was given to Wistar rats and thoracic aortae were dissected 5h later. Nitric oxide spin trapping studies (with Fe-diethyldithiocarbamate) and immunoblot analysis of inducible nitric oxide synthase were performed in media and in adventitia separately. Electron paramagnetic resonance spectra were recorded in an x-band spectrometer Bruker 300E at 77K.

It was found that in aortae treated with lipopolysaccharide *in vitro*, the adventitia generated about 6 times more nitric oxide than in the media (13.1±1.8 versus 2.2±0.2 pmol/μgDNA/h; P<0.01). Immunoblot analysis of inducible nitric oxide synthase also showed more intense signal in the adventitia than in the media. In *ex vivo* studies, nitric oxide production in adventitia and in media were comparable (0.3±0.3 and 0.4±0.2 pmol/μgDNA/h, respectively).

These results provide evidence for the existence of adventitial source of nitric oxide, which can be triggered by lipopolysaccharide both in vitro and in vivo. This adventitia-derived NO may have potential impact on the contractile function of the vessels.

076

cGMP- AND cAMP-DEPENDENT VASODILATORS INHIBIT THE EXPRESSION OF THE CELL CYCLE PROTEINS CYCLIN D1 AND A IN CULTURED VASCULAR SMOOTH MUSCLE CELLS (VSMC)

N. Kronemann, W.A. Nockher, R. Busse, V.B. Schini-Kerth
Centers of Cardiovascular Physiology and Nephrology, University Clinic of Frankfurt, D-60590 Frankfurt am Main, Germany

Cyclins control the transition between the phases of the cell cycle as regulatory subunits of the cyclin-dependent kinases. The aim of the present study was to characterize the antiproliferative effect of cGMP and cAMP-dependent vasodilators, by studying their effects on the progression of cells through the cell cycle and the expression of cyclins.

Cell cycle analysis was assessed by FACScan flow cytometry, and the expression of cyclins by Western blot analysis using quiescent confluent rat aortic smooth muscle cells.

Sodium nitroprusside (SNP) and forskolin reduced the fetal calf serum (FCS)-induced increase in cell number, and the cells were growth arrested in the G0/G1 phase of the cell cycle. FCS induced a time-dependent expression of the G1 cyclins, D1 and E, and the S phase cyclin A. The FCS-induced expression of cyclin D1 and A were significantly reduced by SNP and forskolin whereas that of cyclin E was unaffected. Similar effects were obtained with 8-Br-cGMP and 8-Br-cAMP.

The present findings indicate that nitric oxide donors and cAMP-dependent vasodilators prevent the progression of VSMC from G0/G1 into the S phase of the cell cycle. This effect may be due to a cGMP and cAMP-dependent inhibition of the expression of the cell cycle regulatory proteins cyclin D1 and A.

077

CHARACTERISATION OF VASORELAXATION TO THE SUPEROXIDE ANION SCAVENGER TEMPOL IN VITRO

D.W. Laight, A.V. Kaw, M.J. Carrier, E.E. Änggård
The William Harvey Research Institute, Charterhouse Square, London, EC1M 6BQ, England.

We investigated the role of the endogenous nitric oxide pathway in vasorelaxation to the superoxide anion scavenger TEMPOL (4-hydroxy-2,2,6,6-tetramethylpiperidine-1-oxyl) in rat vascular smooth muscle.

Thoracic aortic rings from male Wistar rats (250-300 g) were mounted in Krebs-Henseleit solution containing indomethacin (10μM) gassed with carbogen and warmed to 37°C. Vasorelaxation to TEMPOL (1-300μM) was assessed after precontraction with noradrenaline (100nM). Some rings were treated with N^G-nitro-L-arginine methyl ester (0.3mM) or the guanylyl cyclase inhibitor ODQ (10μM) while others were denuded of endothelium. Vasorelaxation to TEMPOL (pD_2=5.73±0.06, E_{max}=20.9±6.2%, n=5) occurred over a range compatible with its superoxide anion scavenging activity (Laight et al. Brit J Pharmacol; 119: 237P). Further vasorelaxation could be achieved by acetylcholine (1μM) (78.9±3.1%) and papaverine (100%) (n=5). In contrast, vasorelaxation to TEMPOL was abolished by endothelial denudation and both nitric oxide synthase and guanylyl cyclase inhibition (n=5). Vasorelaxation to acetylcholine (1μM) was abolished in endothelium-denuded rings and reduced to 7.6±2.8% and 8.2±2.0% after treatment with N^G-nitro-L-arginine methyl ester and ODQ, respectively, while papaverine could still elicit 100% vasorelaxation (n=5).

In conclusion, vasorelaxation to TEMPOL in vitro is consistent with an augmentation in basal nitric oxide-mediated vasodilation due to the protection of nitric oxide from inactivation by superoxide anion.

This work was supported by Lipha s.a., Lyon, France.

078

NITRIC OXIDE-MEDIATED VASODILATION IN A MODEL OF OXIDANT STRESS IN VITRO

D.W. Laight, A.V. Kaw, M.J. Carrier, E.E. Änggård
The William Harvey Research Institute, Charterhouse Square, London, EC1M 6BQ, England.

We assessed vasorelaxation to the novel phosphodiesterase type V inhibitor ONO-1505 (4-[2-(2-hydroxyethoxy)ethylamino]-2-(1H-imidazol-1-yl)-6-methoxyquinazoline) (Laight et al. Brit J Pharmacol 1996; 119: 130P) as a marker of basal endothelial function in a model of oxidant stress in isolated rat vascular smooth muscle.

Thoracic aortic rings from male Wistar rats (250-300 g) were mounted in Krebs-Henseleit solution containing indomethacin (10μM) gassed with carbogen and warmed to 37°C. Rings treated with the Cu-Zn superoxide dismutase inhibitor diethyldithiocarbamate (10 mM) for 30 min followed by 30 min washout or sham-treated rings were then equivalently precontracted with noradrenaline (30-100nM) to assess vasorelaxation to ONO-1505 (0.1-10μM), acetylcholine (1nM-1μM) or S-nitroso-N-acetylpenicillamine (0.03-30μM). Vasorelaxation to ONO-1505 (control area under curve=46.8±7.3, n=5) was inhibited (area under curve=20.6±4.0, n=5; P<0.01) while vasorelaxation to acetylcholine and S-nitroso-N-acetylpenicillamine was unaffected. Furthermore, contraction to noradrenaline (1nM-1μM) (control area under curve=2.3±0.2, n=4) was enhanced by diethyldithiocarbamate (area under curve=3.1±0.3, n=4; P<0.05). This effect was abolished by N^G-nitro-L-arginine methyl ester (0.3mM, n=5).

In conclusion, diethyldithiocarbamate treatment resulted in a selective lesion in basal nitric oxide-mediated vasodilation in the rat aorta in vitro. This may reflect endothelial dysfunction due to superoxide anion stress.

This work was supported by Lipha s.a., Lyon, France.

079

ALTERED CHLORIDE (Cl) PERMEABILITY OR DISTRIBUTION EFFECTS CONTRACTIONS TO NOREPINEPHRINE (NE).

F.S. Lamb and T.J. Barna
Dept. of Pediatrics, University of Iowa, Iowa City, Iowa, USA 52242

Cl is concentrated intracellularly in vascular smooth muscle (VSM) producing an equilibrium potential (E_{Cl}) which is 20-30 mV more positive than resting Vm. Increases in Cl conductance (gCl) therefore produce depolarization. We hypothesized that if Cl currents contribute to agonist-induced depolarization, altering E_{Cl} or gCl should alter isometric contractile responses of isolated rat aortic rings. In previous studies we have shown that low Cl buffer (8 mM) substituted with an inpermeant anion (methanesulfonate, MS) increases the initial peak (3 min) contraction to norepinephrine (NE). In contrast, substitution with other anions suppresses contraction (MS 45.5 ± 3.5%, Cl 19.4 ± 2.6%, Bromide 14.3 ± 4.6, Iodide 6.7 ± 4.3% of response to 120 mM KCl). Peak NE-induced contraction was blocked by inhibition of Na-K-2Cl cotransport with 10 µM bumetanide (control 79 ± 9.8%, treated 53 ± 8.3%, n=5) or Cl-HCO3 exchange with 10 mM HEPES buffer (control 80.6 ± 6.2%, treated 39.8 ± 6.9%, n=5). These two effects were additive (control 83.3 ± 8.6%, bumetanide. + HEPES 23 ± 6.7%). These interventions had no effect on contractions to KCl. Cl channel blockers were also tested for their ability to inhibit NE-induced contraction. DIDS (1 mM, 79%, n=5), A-9-C (1 mM, 80%, n=5) and Niflumic acid (100 µM, 68%, n=5) all inhibited ED_{80} NE responses while Tamoxifen (10 µM) did not. Of the three compounds which inhibited NE-induced contraction, only DIDS was completely without effect on KCl-induced contractions. We conclude that a Cl channel with permeability sequence of I>Br>Cl>MS contributes to NE-induced depolarization of rat aorta.

080

CHLORIDE (Cl) ION CURRENTS MODULATE THE RESPONSE OF RAT AORTIC RINGS TO NOREPINEPHRINE (NE).

F.S. Lamb and T.J. Barna
Dept. of Pediatrics, University of Iowa, Iowa City, Iowa, USA 52242

In vascular smooth muscle (VSM), Cl is transported intracellularly producing an equilibrium potential (E_{Cl}) which is more positive than Vm. Increasing Cl conductance therefore produces depolarization. We hypothesized that if Cl currents contribute to resting Vm or agonist-induced depolarization, changing E_{Cl} should alter contractility. Substitution of extracellular Cl with an inert, impermeant anion (methanesulfonate) shifts E_{Cl} to a more positive value. In intact rat aortic rings there is little or no response to low Cl (8mM) buffer (0-3% of response to 120 mM KCl). In endothelial denuded (rubbed) rings a consistent contractile response of variable size is observed (3min 0-82%, 20 min 6-104%, n=9). L-NNA (100 µM) treated rings also contract in low Cl (3 min 80 ± 11%, 20 min 52 ± 30%, n=2). The contractions are completely inhibited by nifedipine (1 µM). In intact rings, an ED_{20} dose of NE produces an initial peak (3 min) and a maintained (20 min) response (3 min 20.5 ± 3.4%, 20 min 13.9 ± 2.7 %). When rings were exposed to low Cl and NE simultaneously responses were potentiated (3 min 52.1 ± 5.9%, 20 min 24.6 ± 4.4%, n=9, $p<0.05$). This effect was Cl concentration-dependent. KCl contractions were unaltered by low Cl. Rubbing augmented the effect of low Cl (control 3 min 16.0 ± 2.0%, 20 min 23.4 ± 3.3%, low Cl peak 86.2 ± 10.2%, 20 min 103.6 ± 14.7%, n=5). Similar results were obtained with L-NNA treatment. The effect of low Cl is blocked by DIDS (1 mM). We conclude: 1) Cl currents contribute to resting Vm 2) a Cl current is important for NE-induced depolarization, 3) either NE-induced endothelial NO' production is Cl current-dependent or NO' suppresses Cl permeability of VSM.

081

EFFECTS OF DIETARY L-ARGININE ON STRUCTURE AND FUNCTION OF FLOW-RESTRICTED VEIN GRAFTS

M. E. Landis, P. Gloviczki and V. M. Miller
Departments of Surgery and Physiology and Biophysics, Mayo Clinic and Foundation, Rochester, MN, USA

Experiments were designed to assess the effect of dietary supplementation with L-arginine on function of vein grafts under conditions of compromised blood flow. Adult male dogs were fed supplemental L-arginine (200 mg/kg/day) one week prior to and following placement of bilateral reversed interposition saphenous vein grafts in femoral arteries. Flow was reduced unilaterally in one graft by 50%. A second group of dogs (control) underwent the identical surgical procedure but did not receive supplemental L-arginine. Four weeks postoperatively, steady state plasma L-arginine concentrations increased from 140 to 153 µM/L; peak serum concentrations of L-arginine occurred within two hours after feeding and were approximately three times greater than baseline levels. In rings of graft suspended for measurement of isometric force, maximal contractions to KCl (60 mM) and relaxations to nitric oxide reduced in grafts from L-arginine-fed dogs. Histologic analysis showed increased cellularity in both control and flow-restricted grafts from arginine-fed compared to control dogs. Results suggest that dietary arginine alters function and structure of flow restricted vein grafts which could affect long-term patency of the grafts.

082

RELATIONSHIP BETWEEN NITRIC OXIDE PRODUCTION AND CYTOSOLIC Ca^{2+} CONCENTRATION IN ENDOTHELIAL CELLS

F. Lantoine, L. Iouzalen, E. Millanvoye van Brussel, M.A. Devynck, M. David-Dufilho
Pharmacology, URA CNRS 1482, University of Paris V, 156 rue de Vaugirard, 75015 Paris, France

Endothelial cells respond to various stimuli by increasing cytosolic Ca^{2+} concentration ($[Ca^{2+}]_i$) and secreting substances which regulate hemostasis and vascular tone. Nitric oxide (NO) is a potent vasodilator and an inhibitor of platelet aggregation. Our purpose was to investigate the role of the transmembrane Ca^{2+} gradient on NO production by real-time measurement of its release from cultured human umbilical vein endothelial cells. NO was detected by differential pulse amperometry with a carbon fiber coated with nickel porphyrin and Nafion films. $[Ca^{2+}]_i$ was measured with fura-2.

Histamine induced NO production and a biphasic $[Ca^{2+}]_i$ rise: a peak reflecting Ca^{2+} release from internal stores followed by a plateau corresponding to Ca^{2+} influx. The suppression of the transmembrane Ca^{2+} gradient or the pre-treatment with 30 µM SK&F 96365, a putative inhibitor of receptor-activated Ca^{2+} influx, abolished both NO production and sustained Ca^{2+} elevation but did not modify the initial Ca^{2+} peak. Similar effects were observed on NO production and Ca^{2+} movements induced by thapsigargin, a specific inhibitor of endoplasmic reticulum Ca^{2+}-ATPase, which increased $[Ca^{2+}]_i$ by activating Ca^{2+} influx without receptor activation. In contrast, the SK&F 96365-induced $[Ca^{2+}]_i$ rises, which only reflected Ca^{2+} release from intracellular stores, were not accompanied by detectable NO production.

These results demonstrate the major role of Ca^{2+} influx in the synthesis of endothelial nitric oxide.

083

ENDOTHELIUM-DEPENDENT RESPONSES TO ACETYLCHOLINE IN THE PORCINE ISOLATED PULMONARY ARTERY.

R.N. Lawrence, W.R. Dunn and V.G. Wilson
Department of Physiology and Pharmacology, Queens Medical Centre, Nottingham, NG7 2UH, UK.

Our aim was to examine the nature of the response to acetylcholine in the porcine isolated pulmonary artery. Segments of the arteries were set up for isometric tension recording. Tissues were precontracted with the thromboxane-mimetic, U46619 (10^{-9} to $3x10^{-8}$M) to 80-120% of the maximum response to 60mmol/L KCl. Concentration-response curves to acetylcholine were then obtained in the absence or presence of (i) the nitric oxide synthase inhibitor, N^G-nitro-L-arginine methyl ester (L-NAME - 100µM); (ii) the cyclooxygenase inhibitor, flurbiprofen (1µM); or (iii) L-NAME and flurbiprofen.

Acetylcholine produced concentration- and endothelium-dependent relaxations (n=6), which were unaffected by 1µM flurbiprofen (n=11; control: pD_2 6.66±0.22, E_{max} 66.7±9.2%; flurbiprofen: pD_2 6.84±0.15, E_{max} 72.4±9.5%). 100µM L-NAME abolished relaxations to acetylcholine which subsequently produced a contraction. This contraction was abolished by flurbiprofen (n=9; at 1µM acetylcholine, % of U46619-induced tone with L-NAME alone was 129.3±11.2 compared to 97.4±7.8 with L-NAME and flurbiprofen). In conclusion, acetylcholine produced endothelium-dependent relaxations in the porcine isolated pulmonary artery which were solely due to the release of nitric oxide. Following inhibition of the nitric oxide pathway, however, acetylcholine elicited contractions, which appear to involve a contractile prostanoid.

084

PEROXYNITRITE PRESERVES MYOCARDIAL INTEGRITY IN VIVO BY INHIBITING LEUKOCYTE-ENDOTHELIAL INTERACTION

Allan M. Lefer
Department of Physiology, Jefferson Medical College of T.J.U.
1020 Locust Street, Philadelphia, PA 19107-6799, U.S.A.

Peroxynitrite ($ONOO^-$), a free radical produced by the interaction of nitric oxide (NO and superoxide, is purported to exert cytotoxic effects in a variety of systems at concentrations ranging from 300 µM to 1.5 mM. However, these concentrations of $ONOO^-$ are unlikely to exist in vivo. Perfusion of $ONOO^-$ at 400 nM directly into the cat heart was accomplished after 80 minutes of a 90 minute ischemia followed by 270 min of reperfusion (MI/R). This concentration of $ONOO^-$ did not exert any effects on blood pressure, heart rate or their product. However, $ONOO^-$ treated MI/R cats exhibited an area of necrosis of 14 ± 2 indexed to the area-at-risk compared to 32 ± 3 for those MI/R cats receiving only a pH matched vehicle (p<0.01). Supporting this cardioprotective effect was an improved vasorelaxation of coronary artery rings isolated from $ONOO^-$ treated MI/R cats 85 ± 4% vs 49 ± 5% for vehicle-treated MI/R cats (p<0.01). No difference was observed in vasorelaxant responses to $NaNO_2$. Moreover, PMN adhesion to I/R cat coronary artery endothelium was reduced by 37% in hearts isolated from MI/R cats receiving 400 nM $ONOO^-$ (p<0.02) although this concentration of $ONOO^-$ was below the threshold for vasodilation. In mesenteries subjected to intravital microscopy in vivo, superfusion of the mesentery with 400-800 nM $ONOO^-$ significantly attenuated leukocyte rolling in response to thrombin stimulation from 67 ± 8 to 16 ± 4 WBCs/min (p<0.01) and reduced WBC adherence from 17 ± 2 to 2 ± 1 WBCs/100 µm mesenteric venule length (p<0.01). These effects appear to be due to inhibition of expression of P-selectin on the vascular endothelium as shown by immunohistochemistry. Thus, $ONOO^-$ given in vivo at physiologic concentrations exerts vasculoprotective effects which translate into significant anti-ischemia/reperfusion actions.

085

PEROXYNITRITE ATTENUATES LEUKOCYTE-ENDOTHELIAL CELL INTERACTIONS

David J. Lefer
Department of Molecular and Cellular Physiology, LSU Medical Cente
1501 Kings Highway, Shreveport, LA 71130-3932, U.S.A.

Peroxynitrite ($ONOO^-$) has been implicated as a toxic mediator in the pathogenesis of a number of disease states including myocardial reperfusion injury. We investigated the effects of $ONOO^-$ on leukocyte -endothelial cell interactions in the intact rat mesentery and in isolated, perfused rat hearts subjected to global ischemia and reperfusion with rat neutrophils (PMNs). In the rat mesentery, superfusion with thrombin (0.5 U/ml) caused a dramatic increase in leukocyte rolling from 11±2 to 76±10 WBCs/min and an increase in leukocyte adherence from 3±1 to 20±3 WBCs/100 µm (p<0.001 vs. control rats). $ONOO^-$ (800nM) superfusion reduced thrombin-mediated leukocyte rolling to 13±3 WBCs/min (p<0.02) and adherence to 4±1 WBCs/100 µm (p<0.01) without affecting systemic blood pressure or venular shear rate. In the isolated ischemic heart, infusion of PMNs ($1x10^8$) during reperfusion resulted in a 57±14% recovery (p<0.01 vs. baseline) of left ventricular developed pressure (LVDP) and a significant (p<0.01) rise in cardiac myeloperoxidase (MPO) activity (2.1±0.50 vs 0.3±0.06 in control hearts). Interestingly, treatment with $ONOO^-$ (800nM) resulted in a 93% recovery of LVDP and significant reduction in MPO activity to 0.2±0.07 U/g tissue (both p<0.01 vs. Vehicle). Furthermore, immunostaining of thrombin treated rat mesentery and the ischemic-reperfused rat heart revealed that P-selectin expressed was markedly enhanced and that $ONOO^-$ treatment significantly reduced the surface expression of this endothelial cell adhesion molecule. We conclude that $ONOO^-$ attenuates leukocyte-endothelial cell interactions following acute inflammation.

086

INVOLVEMENT OF PROTEIN KINASE G IN THE RELAXATION INDUCED BY SPECIFIC CYCLIC AMP PHOSPHODIESTERASE (PDE3 & PDE4) INHIBITORS

C. Lugnier, A.E. Eckly-Michel
Laboratoire de Pharmacologie et de Physiopathologie Cellulaires, CNRS URA 600, Université Louis Pasteur de Strabourg, B.P. 24, 67401, Illkirch, France.

The involvement of protein kinase A and protein kinase G in the effects of cyclic AMP-elevating agents on vascular smooth muscle relaxation and ATP-induced calcium signalling ($[Ca^{2+}]_i$) was studied in rat aorta. Cyclic AMP-elevating agents used were a beta-adrenergic agonist (isoprenaline), a PDE3 inhibitor (SK&F 94120) and a PDE4 inhibitor (rolipram). In intact rat aorta, the relaxant effect induced by isoprenaline (0.01-0.3 µM) was decreased by a specific inhibitor of protein kinase A, H-89, whereas a specific inhibitor of protein kinase G, Rp-8Br-cyclic GMPS, was without effect. At 10 µM, isoprenaline produced no change in smooth muscle cell ATP-induced $[Ca^{2+}]_i$. Neither H-89, nor Rp-8Br-cyclic GMPS, did modify this response. These findings suggest that protein kinase A is only involved in the relaxant effect induced by low concentrations of isoprenaline (0.01 to 0.3 µM). The relaxant effects induced by SK&F 94120 and rolipram were inhibited by Rp-8Br-cyclic GMPS with no significant effect of H-89. Rolipram inhibited the ATP-induced increase in $[Ca^{2+}]i$. This effect was abolished by Rp-8Br-cyclic GMPS, whereas H-89 had no significant effect. Our data support a role of both protein kinase A and protein kinase G in cyclic AMP-mediated relaxation in rat aorta depending on the cellular pathway used to increase cyclic AMP level.

This study suggests that protein kinase G is involved in the vascular effects induced by the inhibitors of PDE3 and PDE4. Since we previously showed that PDE3 and PDE4 inhibitors only increased cyclic AMP levels with no change in cyclic GMP level, these data also suggest a cross-activation of protein kinase G by cyclic AMP in rat aorta which may reflect a colocalization of PDE3 and PDE4 with protein kinase G.

087

DIFFERENTIAL EFFECT OF L-NAME ON NORADRENALINE-INDUCED AND NERVE-MEDIATED VASOCONSTRICTION IN RABBIT CUTANEOUS RESISTANCE ARTERIES

J.B. Macmillan, K.M. Smith, K.M. McCulloch and J.C. McGrath
Clinical Research Initiative in Heart Failure, West Medical Building, University of Glasgow, Glasgow G12 8QQ, Scotland

The objective of this study was to examine the effects of L-NAME or nerve-mediated and exogenous noradrenaline-induced vasoconstriction in rabbit arteries. Cutaneous resistance arteries (internal diameter, $L_{0.9}$=241.9=1.2μm, n=37/21 (arteries/animals)) from New Zealand White rabbits (weighing 3.0-4.5 kg) were mounted (2mm length) on a wire myograph in Krebs (at 37°C), bubbled with 95%O_2/5%CO_2 and normalised (Mulvany & Halpern, Circ. Res. 1977; 41:19-26). L-NAME (100μM), a nitric oxide (NO) synthase inhibitor, significantly increased the sensitivity of rabbit cutaneous arteries to exogenous noradrenaline and also significantly reduced the maximal vasodilatation induced by acetylcholine in these arteries. Control frequency-response curves were produced by stimulating the arteries at 4, 8, 16, 32 and 64Hz (0.1ms pulse width, 1 sec. train, at 35V). Analysis of the effects of cocaine, α,β-methylene ATP and prazosin on frequency response curves indicated that the noradrenergic component of the nerve-mediated response is more dominant that the purinergic component at higher frequencies. However, L-NAME had no significant effect on nerve-mediated responses at any of the frequencies measured. We conclude that rabbit cutaneous resistance arteries have an active noradrenaline reuptake system whose inhibition by cocaine potentiates both nerve-mediated and exogenously applied noradrenaline-induced responses. In our studies of exogenous vasoconstriction, L-NAME (100 μM blocked ACh endothelium-dependent vasodilation to acetylcholine and also increased the sensitivity to noradrenaline implying an influence of receptor-released and constitutive NO on noradrenaline-induced vascular contraction. In contrast versus nerve mediated responses L-NAME has no significant effect indicating no influence of constitutive NO in the control of nerve-mediated vasomotor tone in rabbit resistance arteries.

088

ACTIVATION OF TRANSCRIPTION FACTOR NF-κB BY PLATELET-DERIVED GROWTH FACTOR-STIMULATED SUPEROXIDE ANION IN HUMAN AORTIC SMOOTH MUSCLE CELLS

T. Marumo, V. B. Schini-Kerth, B. Fisslthaler, R. Busse,
Zentrum der Physiologie, Klinikum der Johann Wolfgang Goethe Universität, Theodor-Stern-Kai 7, D-60590 Frankfurt am Main, Germany

Platelet-derived growth factor (PDGF) and superoxide anion have been implicated in the pathogenesis of atherosclerosis. We investigated whether PDGF stimulates the production of superoxide anion in human aortic smooth muscle cells (HSMC), and whether superoxide anion activates nuclear factor-κB (NF-κB) and in this way induces monocyte chemoattractant protein 1 (MCP-1) in PDGF-treated cells.

PDGF-AB (10 - 100 ng/ml) and PDGF-BB (30 and 100 ng/ml), but not PDGF-AA (up to 100 ng/ml) stimulated superoxide anion generation in HSMC, which was attenuated by the NAD(P)H oxidase inhibitor iodonium diphenyl (10 μM), the protein kinase C inhibitor Ro 31-8220 (1 μM), and PI3-kinase inhibitor wortmannin (0.1 μM). Allopurinol (100 μM) and nifedipine (1 μM) had no effect on PDGF-induced superoxide anion generation, while indomethacin (10 μM) potentiated this response. Gel mobility shift assay revealed that PDGF-AB increased the binding activity of NF-κB, which contained predominantly the p50/p65 heterodimer in nuclear extracts from HSMC. PDGF-enhanced NF-κB activation and MCP-1 mRNA induction were inhibited by SOD (500 U/ml) , iodonium diphenyl, Ro 31-8220 and wortmannin.

The results demonstrate that PDGF stimulates superoxide anion generation in HSMC via PKC-dependent and wortmannin-sensitive pathways involving flavoenzyme(s). This PDGF-induced superoxide anion production may be involved in the process of atherogenesis by mediating, at least partly, NF-κB activation and MCP-1 induction.

089

IN VIVO EFFECTS OF OXIDIZED LOW-DENSITY LIPOPROTEIN ON INTIMAL THICKENING AND ENDOTHELIUM-MEDIATED DILATATION

K.E. Matthys, C.E. Van Hove, I.S. Geerts, [#]M.M. Kockx, [*]L.J. Andries, N. Van Osselaer, A.G. Herman, H. Bult
Div. Pharmacol. (UIA) and [*]Physiol. (RUCA), Univ. Antwerp, and [#]Dept. Pathol., Middelheim Hosp., 2610 Wilrijk, Belgium

Based on in vitro studies, oxidized low-density lipoprotein (oxLDL) has been implicated in atherogenesis. The aim of this study was to investigate the effect of in vivo exposure to oxLDL on intimal thickening and relaxing behaviour. Intimal thickening was evoked by a silicone collar placed around the rabbit carotid artery for 2 weeks and oxLDL (Cu^{2+}-oxidized) was delivered to the collar via a subdermally implanted osmotic minipump (7 μg/h in PBS).

The collar induced a discrete intimal hyperplasia (intima/media (I/M) ratio 11 ± 2%). OxLDL application greatly enhanced the intimal thickness (I/M ratio 98 ± 16%). Collaring alone did not impair endothelium-dependent relaxations to acetylcholine. However, decreased sensitivity was observed after exposure to oxLDL (-logEC_{50} oxLDL 6.95 ± 0.11 vs. 7.52 ± 0.11 collar alone) and the maximal relaxation was reduced by 50%, this in the presence of a virtually intact endothelium (CD31 staining). Complete relaxation was observed with the nitric oxide donors glyceryl trinitrate and S-nitroso-N-acetylpenicillamine. Local infusion of lysophosphatidylcholine (0.1-5 nmol/h) did not mimic the effects of oxLDL.

In summary, we demonstrated that vascular exposure to oxLDL in vivo induces similar morphological and functional changes as described in atherosclerotic blood vessels, thereby supporting an active role for oxLDL in lesion formation in vivo.

090

VASODILATOR MECHANISMS IN HEART FAILURE: RESISTANCE ARTERIES IN A RABBIT MODEL AND HUMAN PATIENTS.

J.C. McGrath, E. Beattie, J.G.F. Cleland, P.J. Cowburn, H.J. Dargie, C. Hillier, J.B. Macmillan, J.J.V. McMurray, J.J. Morton & K.M. Smith.
Clinical Research Initiative in Heart Failure, University of Glasgow, Glasgow G12 8QQ, Scotland.

Vascular changes accompanying heart failure may involve vasodilatatory processes such as attenuation of agonist-activated endothelial nitric oxide release or smooth muscle cell signalling. We have now investigated the acetylcholine-mediated vasodilation (noradrenaline 1μM) in resistance arteries from heart failure patients and from a coronary-ligated rabbit model. Cutaneous resistance arteries from New Zealand White rabbits with a left anterior descending coronary artery ligation for 8, 16 or 32 weeks or from buttock biopsies from heart failure patients (and sham-operated or age and sex matched controls) were mounted (2mm length) on a wire myograph. In rabbits, after ligation, the acetylcholine maximum vasodilation was smaller. The vasodilation remaining to acetylcholine after L-NAME (100μM) was greater after ligation: thus the L-NAME-sensitive component was smaller after ligation. This suggests both an attenuation of the NO-dependent component and a possible compensatory increase in other components of acetylcholine's vasodilator action in this heart failure model. No progression of endothelial dysfunction was evident but higher ejection fractions in 32 week survivors indicate less severity. In vessels from heart failure patients maximum vasodilation to acetylcholine, though not to sodium nitroprusside, was smaller than in controls suggesting a deficit at endothelial level. Vasodilator sensitivity to cicaprost was also smaller than in controls suggesting a deficit in vasodilator capacity at the smooth muscle level, possibly related to cAMP rather than cGMP. The study provides new insights to vasodilatory deficits in heart failure, suggests more than a simple deficit in endothelial nitric oxide and points to further changes in endothelial and vascular smooth muscle function in human heart failure which are reflected in the rabbit model.

091

ENDOTHELIAL NITRIC OXIDE SYNTHASE AND SUPEROXIDE DISMUTASE IN A MODEL OF GENETIC HYPERTENSION

M. McIntyre, M.J. Brosnan, C.A. Hamilton, J.L. Reid, A.F. Dominiczak
University Department of Medicine & Therapeutics, Western Infirmary, Glasgow G11 6NT, U.K.

We have previously shown that aortas from stroke prone spontaneously hypertensive rats (SHRSP) have reduced basal vasodilator effect of nitric oxide compared to Wistar-Kyoto (WKY), despite increased endothelial nitric oxide synthase (eNOS) activity. We aimed to determine if SHRSP are deficient in superoxide dismutase (SOD) resulting in increased superoxide accumulation.

Thoracic aortas from 4 WKY females, 4 WKY males, 4 SHRSP females and 3 SHRSP males were removed, cleaned and snap frozen in liquid nitrogen. RNA was extracted by RNAzol B. 10μg of total RNA was run on a 1.2% agarose gel, blotted onto Hybond N membrane and hybridised with probes for glyceraldehyde phosphate dehydrogenase (GAPDH), manganese (Mn) SOD and copper/zinc (Cu/Zn) SOD.

The MnSOD/GAPDH ratio (±SEM) in SHRSP (0.69±0.05) is significantly greater than WKY males (0.32±0.01)(95% CI -0.58, -0.15; p=0.02). There were no significant strain differences in MnSOD in females (95% CI -1.11, 0.12; p=0.09) or Cu/ZnSOD in males (95% CI -0.98, 2.82; p=0.22) or females (95% CI -0.74, 0.17; p=0.14).

We conclude that SHRSP are not deficient in SOD. Indeed, SHRSP males have greater MnSOD expression. We speculate that increased superoxide anion production is the primary abnormality responsible for endothelial dysfunction in SHRSP, whereas expression of eNOS and MnSOD may be upregulated as a compensatory mechanism.

092

ANTICONSTRICTOR EFFECT OF SHEAR STRESS-INDUCED SMOOTH MUSCLE RELAXATION

A.M. Melkumyants, S.P. Kartamyshev, S.A. Balashov
National Cardiology Research Center, 121552, Moscow, Russia

In acute experiments on anesthetized cats we assessed the effect of endothelium-dependent shear stress-induced smooth muscle relaxation on noradrenaline-induced constriction of femoral vascular bed. Changes in resistance of proximal arterial vessels (arteries and large arterioles) caused by noradrenaline ($2 \cdot 10^{-7}$ M, ia) during perfusion of the hindlimb under a constant blood flow or a constant pressure before and after endothelium impairment were compared. Since the shear stress is directly related to blood flow and inversely related to the third power of vessel diameter, it rises at vasoconstriction under a constant blood flow thus evoking smooth muscle relaxation. Under a constant perfusion pressure, vasoconstriction is accompanied by a decrease in flow rate that prevents the wall shear stress increase. The comparison of the responses at these two regimes permits to reveal anticonstrictor effect of shear stress-induced dilation.

We found that in endothelium-intact vessels noradrenaline-induced increase of proximal arterial resistance at a constant flow was 5.3±0.4 times smaller than at a constant pressure perfusion. Removal of the endothelium enhanced the responses at a constant flow 4.7±0.4-fold, while vasoconstriction at a constant pressure increased by only 12%. Selective blockade of the endothelium sensitivity to shear stress (that was achieved by 30 s perfusion of the bed with saline containing 0.02% glutaraldehyde dimer) augmented constriction at a constant flow 4.6±0.3-fold, without any effect on the responses at a constant pressure. These data demonstrate that, at a constant blood flow, shear stress-induced smooth muscle relaxation is the most powerful endothelium-mediated factor opposing constriction caused by noradrenaline.

093

THE ANTI-MULTIDRUG RESISTANCE AGENT S9788 IS A POTENT VASODILATOR.

Jean-Vivien Mombouli, Rajy Matthews and Josette Veve.
Center for Experimental Therapeutics, Baylor College of Medicine, Houston, TX 77030, USA.

Experiments were designed to determine whether or not S9788 causes vasodilatation in vitro in isolated arteries. In conventional organ chamber experiments, rings from isolated rat mesenteric and canine coronary arteries were suspended in oxygenated physiological solution. The tissues were contracted with agonists or elevated K solutions, to examine the effects of S9788 on receptor- and depolarization-induced contractions of vascular smooth muscle, respectively. S9788 did not induce contractions both in rat and canine arteries. In the rat mesenteric artery without endothelium, S9788 caused concentration-relaxation curves in both receptor- and depolarization-induced contractions of vascular smooth muscle. The effect of S9788 was not readily reversible under our experimental conditions. In canine coronary arteries with and without endothelium, S9788 caused relaxation that was not affected by either the removal of the endothelium, inhibition of NO and/or prostanoid synthesis. S9788 induced relaxation of receptor- and depolarization-induced contractions of coronary arterial smooth muscle with the same potency, under all experimental conditions. These relaxations developed very slowly, in contrast to the rat mesenteric artery. In permeabilized rat mesenteric arteries, S9788 inhibited the Ca^{2+}-induced activation of the contractile machinery. The results show that S9788 causes an endothelium-independent relaxation of vascular smooth muscle at clinically relevant concentrations. Beyond inhibition of the influx of Ca^{2+}, these results show that S9788 interferes with the activation of the contractile machinery by Ca^{2+}. The slow kinetics of the response in the larger mammal suggest that the hypotensive action of S9788 would be difficult to titrate in the clinical setting.

094

NOVEL MECHANISM OF POTENTIATION OF KININS BY INHIBITORS OF ANGIOTENSIN CONVERTING ENZYME.

Jean-Vivien Mombouli.
Center for Experimental Therapeutics, Baylor College of Medicine, Houston, TX 77030, USA.

Angiotensin converting enzyme (ACE) inactivates bradykinin, a potent endothelium-dependent vasodilator. The hypothesis that ACE-inhibitors potentiate kinins independently of prevention of their hydrolysis was investigated. Rings of dog coronary artery degraded bradykinin into penta- and heptapeptides, as determined by electrospray tandem mass spectrometry following extraction and desalting of peptides from the supernatant. This hydrolysis was abolished by the ACE-inhibitor perindoprilat. [Hyp^3,$Tyr(Me)^8$]-bradykinin was very slowly degraded by the arteries; an effect blocked by perindoprilat. This indicates that [Hyp^3,$Tyr(Me)^8$]-bradykinin interacts with ACE. Conventional organ chamber experiments, showed that [Hyp^3,$Tyr(Me)^8$]-bradykinin caused endothelium-dependent relaxations like bradykinin. Both kinins triggered the release of NO and EDHF to induce relaxation. Perindoprilat potentiated more the relaxations to [Hyp^3,$Tyr(Me)^8$]-bradykinin. Perindoprilat had no effect on B_2-receptors antagonists, except for a low concentration of [Hyp^3,$DPhe^7$, Leu^8]-bradykinin. The latter suggests that allosteric potentiation by ACE-inhibitors of binding of ligands to kinin receptors is unlikely. After deactivation of ACE with hydroquinosulfonic acid (HQS, a Zn^{2+} chelator), the acute potentiation of [Hyp^3,$DPhe^7$, Leu^8]-bradykinin by perindoprilat was reduced. Actually, HQS alone significantly enhanced the relaxation induced by [Hyp^3,$DPhe^7$, Leu^8]-bradykinin. This suggests that inhibition of the binding of kinins to ACE (a Zn^{2+}-dependent process) by HQS - or perindoprilat -is responsible for the potentiation. Taken together, the data support the novel concept that, in addition to its hydrolytic function, ACE exerts a buffering function for nanomolar concentrations of kinins.

095

MECHANISM OF THE RESISTANCE OF EDHF TO INHIBITORS OF CYTOCHROME P450 AND PHOSPHOLIPASE A_2.

Jean-Vivien Mombouli
Center for Experimental Therapeutics, Baylor College of Medicine, Houston, TX 77030, USA.

Assuming that epoxyeicosatrienoic acids (EETs) account for endothelium-derived hyperpolarizing factor (EDHF), experiments were designed to test the hypothesis that EETs incorporated into phospholipids account for EDHF, and not the newly synthesized epoxides. In canine coronary arteries, endothelium-dependent relaxations to acetylcholine, bradykinin, arachidonic acid thimerosal or A23187 were resistant to inhibition of the synthesis of NO and prostanoids, and thereby attributed in part to EDHF. The phospholipase C inhibitor U73122 abolished the relaxations to bradykinin, but not to the other compounds. The phospholipase A_2 inhibitor AACOCF3 attenuated the relaxations elicited by the kinin, whereas cytochrome P450 inhibitors (e.g. miconazole) are ineffective. However, in the combined presence of AACOCF3 and miconazole a progressive inhibition of the relaxation to repeated stimulation with bradykinin was obtained. Neither blocker alone induced this progressive inhibition. Cascade bioassays showed that EDHF released from carotid arteries is detectable after treating the vessels with acetylcholine and thimerosal. The combination of U73122 (to block the relaxation induced by acetylcholine) with AACOCF3 (to block the relaxation induced by thimerosal) abolished the release of EDHF. Miconazale had no effect on both the action or the release of EDHF from canine carotid arteries. The absence of acute effects of cytochrome P450 inhibitors is consistent with the idea that *de novo* synthesis of EETs does not lead to EDHF-mediated responses in canine arteries. Furthermore, the inhibitory actions of U73122 and AACOCF3 support the existence of a pool of epoxyeicosatrienoyl phospholipids which is mobolized during EDHF-mediated responses. Inhibition of relaxations to arachidonate by P450-inhibitors reflects the impairment of the de novo synthesis of EETs.

096

STIFFNESS OF THE RADIAL ARTERY WALL MATERIAL IN SUBJECTS WITH END-STAGE RENAL DISEASE (ESRD).

JJ Mourad, X Girerd, P Boutouyrie, S Laurent, ME Safar, GM London.
Broussais Hospital and Inserm U337 , 96 rue didot 75014 Paris, France.

Incremental elastic modulus (Einc) is a marker of the stiffness of vascular wall material. In isobaric conditions, Einc is reduced at the site of the radial artery of subjects with essential hypertension (HT) and increased in subjects with ESRD when measured at the site of the carotid artery. Whether the changes in Einc are influenced by the topography of the vessels and/or by the presence of ESRD is largelly ignored.

A population of 19 ESRD patients was compared with a group of hypertensive patients and normotensives controls. Transcutaneous measurements of radial artery internal diameter, wall thickness and digital pressure were performed, allowing to calculate Einc both in operational and isobaric (100 mmHg) conditions on an arterial site devoid of atherosclerosis.

Internal diameter was identical in the 3 groups. Wall thickness and mean blood pressure were significantly increased in subjects with HT but not in ESRD patients. Circumferential wall stress was identical in the 3 groups. For the same operational wall stress, Einc (kPa.10^3) was increased in patients with ESRD (5.53±4.0 versus 3.3±2.4 in controls; $p<.05$) and normal in subjects with essential hypertension (3.87±4.0). In isobaric conditions, Einc was significantly decreased in subjects with hypertension and increased in patients with ESRD. Thus, in patients with ESRD, the stiffness of the radial artery wall material is increased and the demonstrated alterations of the arterial wall are independant on the level of blood pressure and tensile stress.

097

PHYSIOLOGY OF PROSTACYCLIN (PGI2) AND THROMBOXANE (TxA2): STATE OF THE ART

VUJADIN M.MUJOVIĆ, TOMISLAV JOVANOVIĆ, ŽIVAN MAKSIMOVIĆ and NINOSLAV RADOVANOVIĆ

Intitute of Physiology, School of Medicine, Belgrade, Yugoslavia

University clinic of Cardiovascular surgery. Novi Sad

Extensive studies for the last decade have shown the biological significance of prostaglandins and other eicosanoid in body homeostasis. It is now established without doubt that endothelial cells play a key role in the control of vascular functions and the protective role of the endothelium against vasospasm and unwanted coagulation of the blood. Endothelial prostacyclin (PGI2) is the most potent endogenons vasodilatator and inhibitor of platelet aggregation yet discovered, the actions of which oppose those of TxB2 from platelet. It has several physiological functions but many of them still under intensive research. We have recently reported that PGI2/TxA2 imbalance may be an important determinant of platelet vessel interaction which are vital in circulatory homeostasis. We have been using the original protocol for Na PGI2 treatment of 70 patients with clinical stages III and IV of peripheral arterial occlusive disease (PAOD), and in more than 1000 patients following coronary bypass suregery and total endarterectomy. Na-PGI2, epoprostenol infusion was applied in dose of 5 ng/kg/min for about 16 hours. We conclude that PGI2 is a powerful vasodilator and has beneficially actions in patients with PAOD as well as in vasospasam prevention after myocardial revascularisation and reperfusion respectivaly.

098

N-ACETYLCYSTEINE SENSITIVE NITRIC OXIDE STORAGE IN LIPOPOLYSACCHARIDE-TREATED RAT AORTA

B. Muller, A. Kleschyov, S. Malblanc, J.C Stoclet
Laboratoire de Pharmacologie, CNRS URA 600, F-67401 Illkirch cedex.

We have previously reported the formation of protein-bound dinitrosyl-iron complexes in lipopolysaccharide-treated rat aorta and provided evidence that thiols such as N-acetylcysteine may interfere with these complexes (to generate low molecular weight dinitrosyl-iron species) and produce relaxation. In this study, we further investigated the mechanism of the N-acetylcysteine induced relaxation.

Rat aortic rings were incubated for 18 h in the absence or in the presence of lipopolysaccharide (10 µg/ml) and L-arginine (1 mM). After this period, isometric tension was recorded. In rings incubated with lipopolysaccharide (but not in controls), N-acetylcysteine (0.1 to 10 mM) produced a relaxation which was completely abolished by the guanylyl-cyclase inhibitors methylene blue (3 µM) or oxadiazoloquinoxalin-1-one (1 µM). This relaxation was not associated with an increase of cyclic GMP content in aortic rings. Tetrabutylammonium (3 mM, as a non selective K^+ channel inhibitor) or KCl (50 mM) significantly attenuated the relaxation induced by N-acetylcysteine, whereas glibenclamide, charybdotoxin, apamin or 4-aminopyridine were ineffective. In another set of experiments, the effect of exogenous low molecular weight dinitrosyl-iron complexes (1 nM to 10 µM) was investigated. These complexes produced an endothelium-independent relaxation which was antagonized by methylene blue or oxadiazoloquinoxalin-1-one and was associated with an increase of cyclic GMP content. The relaxation produced by exogenous dinitrosyl-iron complexes was unaffected by tetrabutylammonium or KCl.

Altogether, these results show that in lipopolysaccharide-treated rat aorta, N-acetylcysteine produces a relaxation via cyclic GMP-independent mechanism which probably involves the activation of K^+ channels. However, they do not support the idea that dinitrosyl-iron complexes released by N-acetylcysteine serve as a carrier between nitric oxide stores and guanylyl-cyclase.

099

ADENOSINE INDUCED HYPERPOLARIZATION IN GUINEA-PIG CORONARY ARTERY INVOLVES A_{2b} RECEPTORS AND K_{ATP} CHANNELS

V.N.Mutafova-Yambolieva, K.D.Keef
Department of Physiology & Cell Biology, University of Nevada, Anderson Medical Sciences Building/352, Reno, Nevada 89557-0046

Adenosine (ADO) is known to induce vasodilation and to activate K_{ATP} channels in vascular smooth muscle but the mechanism underlying these effects remains controversial. In the present study employing conventional intracellular microelectrode technique ADO (1-100 µM) elicited concentration dependent hyperpolarization in the guinea-pig coronary artery (EC_{50} 7.5±0.5 µM) which averaged 28.6±3.0 mV at 100 µM ADO. The A_1 selective agonist N^6-cyclopenthyladenosine (CPA), the A_1/A_2 agonist 2-chloroadenosine (2-CADO), and the A_{2a} / A_{2b} receptor activator NECA, 10µM, induced glybenclamide (3 µM) - sensitive hyperpolarization. However, two different selective A_{2a} receptor agonists, i.e., CGS 21680 and DPMA were without effect. The effects of both CPA and NECA were significantly reduced by the specific adenylyl cyclase (AC) inhibitor SQ 22,539 (100 µM). Activation of the AC/cAMP pathway by three other methods i.e., i) forskolin (0.3-1 µM), ii) isoproterenol (0.1-1 µM) and iii) combined milrinone (0.4 µM) and rolipram (30 µM), also gave rise to glybenclamide-sensitive hyperpolarization. Three site-specific activators of type I and type II PKA (i.e., 6-Phe-cAMP, 8-AHA-cAMP, and Sp-5,6-DCl-cBIMPS; 100 µM) hyperpolarized cells in a glybenclamide-sensitive manner, as well.

These results suggest that adenosine hyperpolarizes the membrane via stimulation of A_{2b} receptors which activate AC. Cyclic AMP then activates PKA which increases the activity of K_{ATP} channels. Our results further suggest that K_{ATP} channels are an important target for numerous pathways which raise cAMP levels in the coronary artery.

Supported by NIH grant HL 40399.

100

HYPERPOLARIZATION AND RELAXATION OF CANINE VASCULAR SMOOTH MUSCLE TO VASOACTIVE INTESTINAL POLYPEPTIDE

M. Nakashima, and P. M. Vanhoutte
Surgical Center, Saga Medical School, Saga 849, Japan, and Center for Experimental Therapeutics, Baylor College of Medicine, Houston, Texas, U.S.A.

Vasoactive intestinal polypeptide (VIP) induces relaxation and hyperpolarization of isolated blood vessels. The influence of the endothelium on the response to VIP depends both upon the species and the blood vessel studied. The present study was designed to determine the influence of the endothelium on the hyperpolarization induced by VIP in smooth muscle cells of canine blood vessels, and the potential contribution that these electrophysiological changes may make to the relaxant effects of VIP. Membrane potential was measured in isolated canine coronary arteries and saphenous veins, using glass microelectrodes. Isometric force was recorded in a conventional organ chamber. All experiments were performed in the presence of indomethacin. VIP induced concentration-dependent and endothelium-independent hyperpolarization of the saphenous vein. This response was abolished by glibenclamide. VIP did not induce hyperpolarization of coronary arterial smooth muscle either in the presence or absence of the endothelium. VIP caused concentration-dependent and endothelium-independent relaxations of both arterial and venous rings. The relaxation of the saphenous vein to VIP was not influenced by glibenclamide. These data suggest that hyperpolarization of the cell membrane does not play a significant role in the relaxation of canine blood vessels to VIP.

101

PROTEIN TYROSINE KINASE AS A POSSIBLE MECHANO-SENSOR IN THE GENESIS OF THE PRESSURE-INDUCED VASCULAR CONTRACTION

K. Nakayama, N. Masumoto, Y. Tanabe, K. Obara
Department of Pharmacology, Faculty of Pharmaceutical Sciences, University of Shizuoka, 52-1 Yada, Shizuoka 422, Japan.

In order to elucidate the involvement of protein tyrosine kinase(s) in the pressure-induced contraction, we compared the effect of three structurally- unrelated tyrosine kinase inhibitors and orthovanadate, a tyrosine phosphatase inhibitor, on the pressure-induced myogenic contraction of the posterior cerebral artery isolated from rats and rabbits. The change in vessel diameter was continuously measured with arteriograph. Herbimycin A, a benzoquinone ansamycin, specifically inhibited the pressure-induced contraction (IC_{50} = 5.7 nM), while it only slightly affected contractions in response to potassium chloride and a thromboxane A2 analog. Genistein and tyrphostin 23 significantly attenuated contractions produced by three different stimuli, i.e., pressure, depolarization and agonistic vasoconstrictor. Orthovanadate potentiated the pressure- induced contraction, which was effectively eliminated by the pretreatment with herbimycin A. Furthermore, herbimycin A effectively attenuated protein tyrosyl phosphorylation of 200 kD in vascular tissues, including rabbit cerebral and pulmonary artery, in response to pressure stimuli. These results suggest that tyrosine kinases of *src* family and a target of herbimycin A, play an important role as a mechano-sensor in the pressure-induced contraction of vascular tissues.

102

WHAT DOES IMPEDE WORK-INDUCED CAPILLARY GROWTH IN SKELETAL MUSCLE?

T.L.Nemirovskaya,*B.S.Shenkman,V.B.Koshelev
Dept. of Pathophysiology, Moscow State University, 119899 Moscow, Russia and *Institute of Biomedical Problems, Moscow, Russia

Endurance training often induces capillary neoformation in skeletal muscles. But this process soon slows down and capillary per fibre ratio (CF) reaches the plateau (Adolffsson,1986). The purpose of the present study was to investigate what impeded the capillary neoformation. One possibility was that action of exercise stimulus weakened in the course of adaptation, the other one was that some inhibiting factor was accumulated in the muscle. 18 Wistar rats (200-280 g) were subjected to 4 weeks running on treadmill (30 m/min, 35 min/day,5 days/week). Then 6 rats were killed. CF in m.gastrocnemius lateralis in sedentary controls and after 4 weeks training were respectively 0.97±0.10 (n=5) (±SE) and 1.51±0.20 (n=6) ($p<0.05$). Six rats went on training in the previous conditions and six rats with elevated duration of exercise session (70 min/day) for 4 weeks more. After 8 weeks of 35 min/day training CF was 1.59±0.11 (n=6), and after 70 min/day training CF was 1.90±0.11 (n=7) (higher than after 4 weeks' training ($p<0.05$) and higher than after 8 weeks' 35 min/day training ($p<0.07$). It is concluded that it seems no inhibiting factor for capillary growth is present in the trained muscle. The capillary growth is impeded under constant training conditions because the stimulus (or stimuli) may become not sufficient to induce it.

103

PRE - AND POST-JUNCTIONAL MECHANISMS OF ADRENO-MEDULLIN-INDUCED RELAXATION IN CANINE ARTERIES

T. Okamura, N. Toda
Department of Pharmacology, Shiga University of Medical Science, Seta, Ohtsu 520-21, Japan.

Vasodilator action of adrenomedullin (AM) was analysed in isolated canine arteries. The AM-induced relaxation in central retinal arteries was more potent than that in cerebral, coronary, mesenteric, renal or femoral arteries. The relaxation was endothelium-independent and unaffected by indomethacin, N^G-nitro-L-arginine or glibenclamide. Treatment with [8-37] calcitonin gene-related peptide (CGRP) markedly inhibited the relaxation by AM as that by CGRP. High concentration of sodium nitroprusside abolished the relaxation caused by nitroglycerin and atrial natriuretic peptide and reduced the relaxation caused by AM and CGRP. Treatment with a high concentration of beraprost, a stable analog of prostaglandin I_2, suppressed the response to AM and CGRP but not to nitroglycerin.

In perfused isolated canine mesenteric arteries, pressor actions by transmural electrical stimulation were inhibited by AM. The inhibitory potency of AM was greater than that of CGRP or proadrenomedullin NH_2-terminal 20 peptide. [8-37] CGRP did not affect the inhibitory action of AM, but suppressed the CGRP-induced inhibition.

It may be concluded that potent vasodilatation caused by AM is due to both pre- and post-junctional mechanisms; the former is due to the inhibition of adrenergic neuronal transmission without a mediation of $CGRP_1$ receptors and the latter is endothelium-independent relaxation mediated primarily by intracellular cyclic AMP by stimulation of $CGRP_1$ receptors and partly by cyclic GMP.

104

EFFECTS OF ATRIOPEPTIN ON Ca^{2+} AND K^+ CURRENTS OF RABBIT PULMONARY ARTERY MYOCYTES

Oleg N. Osipenko, Alison M. Gurney
Department of Physiology & Pharmacology, University of Strathclyde, Royal College, Glasgow G1 1XW, Scotland, UK.

The effects of extracellular atriopeptin (fragment 5-27, rat atrial natriuretic peptide) application on membrane ionic currents were studied in smooth muscle cells, enzymatically dissociated from rabbit main pulmonary artery, using the whole-cell recording technique at room temperature. In myocytes dialysed with Cs-intracellular solution, atriopeptin (30nM - 3μM) produced partially reversible, dose-dependent decreases of $I_{Ca(L)}$ amplitude at test potentials (TP) between -20 and +40 mV, with IC_{50} near 1μM. Atriopeptin did not shift the voltage-dependence of activation or inactivation of $I_{Ca(L)}$. When cells were dialysed with K-intracellular solution, with or without 1mM GTP and ATP, I_K activated at TP>30 mV was increased 20% by atriopeptin (100nM - 1μM), but not in the presence of 10 mM TEA, implying that it reflected an increase of amplitude of $I_{BK(Ca)}$. At TP of -30 to 10 mV, where $I_{K(V)}$ was dominant, atriopeptin enhanced I_K by 20%, in the absence or presence of TEA. Atriopeptin (1μM) also reduced by 30% the amplitude of the non-inactivating I_K ($I_{K(N)}$, Evans AM Al. J Physiol 1996; 496: 407-420). Glibenclamide (10μM) did not modify the effects of atriopeptin, indicating no effect on $I_{K(ATP)}$. These results suggest that at least three distinct ionic channels (Ca_L, BK_{Ca} and K_V) are simultaneously involved in the vasodilator effect of atriopeptin on pulmonary artery.

Supported by the British Heart Foundation.

105

MODULATION OF CEREBRAL VASCULAR AUTOREGULATION BY POTASSIUM CHANNELS

R. Paterno, F.M. Faraci, D.D. Heistad
University of Iowa, Iowa City, Iowa 52242; Universita di Reggio Calabria, Catanzaro, Italy.

The goal of this study was to determine whether cerebral autoregulation during acute increases in arterial pressure is modulated by activation of K^+ channels. Diameter of cerebral arterioles (baseline = 42±2 μm, mean±SE) was measured in anesthetized rats. Mean arterial pressure (baseline = 118±3 mmHg) was increased by infusion of phenylephrine iv.

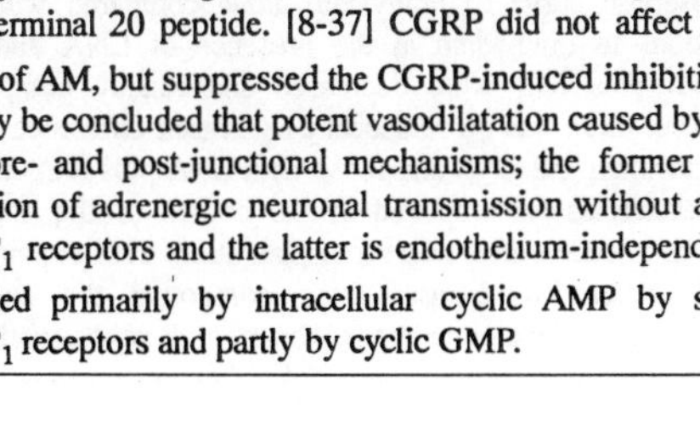

Increases in arteriolar diameter that occurred at high levels of blood pressure were attenuated greatly (P<0.05) by topical 4-aminopyridine (4-AP, 0.2mM), an inhibitor of voltage-dependent K^+ channels (see Graph). Vasoconstrictor responses to U46619 and vasodilator responses to dibutyryl cAMP were not altered by 4-AP. Increases in arteriolar diameter during increases in arterial pressure were also inhibited by iberiotoxin (100 nM, an inhibitor of Ca^{++}-dependent K^+ channels). Thus, K^+ channels may be major modulators of cerebral autoregulation during increases in arterial pressure. Furthermore, "breakthrough" of autoregulation at high levels of pressure may be an active phenomenon.

106

HUMAN GLYCOSYLATED OXYHEMOGLOBIN INDUCES HYPERTROPHY OF RAT AORTIC VASCULAR SMOOTH MUSCLE CELLS IN CULTURE

C. Peiró, E. Madrigal, J. Angulo, J.L. Llergo, L. Rodríguez-Mañas, C.F. Sánchez-Ferrer
Departamento de Farmacología y Terapéutica, Facultad de Medicina, Universidad Autónoma de Madrid, and Unidad de Investigación y Servicio de Geriatría, Hospital Universitario de Getafe, Madrid, Spain

We have demonstrated that highly glycosylated human oxyhemoglobin alters vascular function by impairing endothelium-mediated relaxation (Angulo J et Al. Hypertension 1996; 28: 583-592). The aim of the present study was to assess whether 14%-glycosylated human hemoglobin may produce structural alterations in the vascular wall, particularly at the medial level. Cultured rat aortic vascular smooth muscle cells were treated for 2 days with 14%-glycosylated or non-glycosylated human hemoglobin (1 nM to 1 μM). At the end of the treatment, planar cell surface area was determined by image analysis. Glysolylated hemoglobin induced a concentration-dependent increase in cell size, with threshold concentration of 10 nM and maximal effect at 1 μM (122.4±4.9% and 140.3±5.7% over basal size, respectively). Non-glycosylated hemoglobin significantly increased cell size only at the highest concentration used (113.5±4.4% over basal). Superoxide dismutase (50 to 400 U/ml) abolished the effect of 10 nM glycosylated hemoglobin in a concentration-dependent manner, whereas catalase (100 to 400 U/ml) had no effect. When vascular smooth muscle cells were treated with xanthine (0.1 mM)/xanthine oxidase (1 to 300 μU/ml), as a source of superoxide anions, a concentration-dependent increase in cell size was observed, with maximal effect at 100 μU/ml xanthine oxidase (135.5±7.6% over basal). The effect of xanthine oxidase on cell size was abolished either by 100 μM allopurinol or 200 U/ml superoxide dismutase. We conclude that highly glycosylated human hemoglobin produces vascular smooth muscle cell hypertrophy through the generation of superoxide anions.

107

DECREASE OF $[Ca^{2+}]_i$ BUT NOT HYPERPOLARIZATION IS IMPORTANT FOR DILATION OF RAT CEREBRAL ARTERIES TO ACIDOSIS.

PENG HL, AALKJÆR C
Dept. Pharmacology, University of Aarhus, 8000 Aarhus C, Denmark

Based on the effect of hypercapnic acidosis on isometric tension and membrane potential it has been argued that membrane hyperpolarization is important for the effect of acidosis.

In this study we have tested this idea by assessing the effect of normoacpnic (HCO_3^- reduced from 25 to 8 mM, pH reduced from 7.5 to 7.0) and hypercapnic (CO_2 increased from 5% to 20%, pH reduced from 7.5 to 7.0) acidosis on lumen diameter (isobaric conditions, 40 mmHg and no flow), $[Ca^{2+}{}_i]$ (fura-2) and membrane potential (microelectrodes) of rat middle cerebral arteries. Data give mean±SE for 5 to 8 experiments per group.

Normocapnic and hypercapnic acidosis caused a 40±10 μm and 34±10 μm increase of diameter and a 105±25 nM and 55±12 nM decrease of $[Ca^{2+}]_i$, respectively, which was not significantly different. However, while normocapnic acidosis caused 3.1±1.3 mV depolarization, hypercapnic acidosis caused 6.2±1.7 mV hyperpolarization and these values were significantly different In arteries activated with 50 mM potassium both normocapnic and hypercapnic acidosis caused an increase of diameter (41±12 μm and 28±6 μm, respectively) and a decrease of $[Ca^{2+}]_i$ (158±57 nM and 103±48 nM, respectively).

We conclude that although hypercapnic acidosis causes hyperpolarization, the importance of this hyperpolarization for the vasodilation is unclear since the relaxation and decrease of $[Ca^{2+}]_i$ also was seen in potassium depolarized vessels and since normocapnic acidosis caused a similar vasodilation and decrease of $[Ca^{2+}]_i$ despite membrane depolarization.

108

L-NITRO ARGININE-RESISTANT RELAXATIONS OF CORONARY ARTERIES ARE IMPAIRED AFTER HEART TRANSPLANTATION.

L.P. Perrault, J.P. Bidouard, N. Villeneuve, J.P. Vilaine, and P.M. Vanhoutte.
Institut de Recherches Servier, Suresnes, France.

In a previously described model of heterotopic swine heart transplantation, without initial ischemia-reperfusion injury and without immunosuppression, the endothelial dysfunction due to rejection is selective for Gi-protein mediated relaxations associated with a decreased of nitric oxide availability. The present study was designed to evaluate the integrity of relaxations due to endothelium-derived hyperpolarizing factor (EDHF) after heart transplantation. Vascular reactivity studies of native and allografts epicardial coronary arteries rings six weeks after implantation were performed in standard organ chambers experiments. In the presence of indomethacin and propranolol, the endothelium-dependent relaxations of native coronary arteries to bradykinin were decreased in the presence of L-Nitro Arginine (LNA) and further decreased in the presence of LNA plus potassium chloride (KCl, 20 mmol/L), attesting to the functional presence of EDHF. In allografted coronary arteries, there was a rightward shift of the concentration response curve to bradykinin alone compared with native arteries. Relaxations to bradykinin in the presence of LNA and in the presence of LNA plus KCl were decreased significantly compared to bradykinin alone but there was no statistically significant difference between relaxations to bradykinin and LNA and those with LNA plus KCl. Thus, the LNA-resistant relaxations are impaired in the course of the endothelial dysfunction due to rejection after heart transplantation. This impairment of EDHF-mediated relaxing mechanisms may compound the endothelial dysfunction preceding the development of coronary graft vasculopathy.

109

ENDOTHELIAL DYSFUNCTION AND ATHEROSCLEROSIS IN THE WORKING VERSUS NON-WORKING HETEROTOPIC TRANSPLANTED HEART.

L.P. Perrault, N. Villeneuve, J.P. Bidouard, J.P. Vilaine, and P.M. Vanhoutte.
Institut de Recherches Servier, 11, rue des Moulineaux Suresnes, France.

Shear stress variations, transmyocardial pressure gradients and non laminar blood flow may influence the development of accelerated atherosclerosis by affecting endothelial function and the release of nitric oxide. The purpose of the present study was to compare "non-working" versus "working" porcine heterotopic transplanted hearts models with regard to the development of coronary endothelial dysfunction and intimal hyperplasia. Immunologic typing was performed to allow graft survival with low grade rejection without immunosuppression. Retroperitoneal "non-working" heterotopic transplantations and "working" heart (with left ventricular filling) transplantations were performed. The left ventricular pressure in the non-working group was 0 ± 0 mm Hg and 91 ± 11 mm Hg in the working and the left ventricle to systemic arterial pressure ratio was 0.76 ± 0.08. Sixty days after transplantation, the endothelial function and intimal thickening of coronary epicardial arteries were compared using organ chamber experiments and histological analysis. Both working and non-working allografts developped a comparable selective endothelial dysfunction of G-protein mediated relaxations (relaxations to serotonin and UK14,304 and to sodium fluoride, a direct activator of G-proteins). Relaxations to bradykinin and the calcium ionophore A23187 were unaffected. The prevalence of intimal hyperplasia was 66.1% (117/177) and 68.7% (88/128) in the non-working and working groups, respectively. Thus, working allografts exhibit the same degree and type of endothelial dysfunction and intimal hyperplasia as non working grafts. Nitric oxide release is probably not influenced by the differences in hemodynamics in these two models.

110

DIFFERENT MECHANISMS MEDIATE VASODILATATION TO ENDOTHELIUM-DERIVED NITRIC OXIDE, EXOGENOUS NITRIC OXIDE AND THE NITRIC OXIDE DONOR SIN-1

F. Plane, R. Cohen[1] & C.J. Garland
Department of Pharmacology, University of Bristol, University Walk, Bristol, BS8 1TD, UK and [1] Vascular Biology Unit, Boston University Medical Center, 88E Newton St., Boston 02118, USA.

Acetylcholine-evoked relaxation and repolarisation of the rabbit isolated carotid artery are both mediated by the release of endothelium-derived nitric oxide (Plane F et al. Br J Pharmacol 1996; 117:77P). In the present study, the mechanisms underlying relaxation to acetylcholine, exogenous nitric oxide and the nitric oxide donor SIN-1 in isolated segments of the rabbit carotid artery were investigated further.

SIN-1 (0.1-10 μM), acetylcholine (0.03-10 μM) and exogenous nitric oxide(0.01-10 μM) evoked concentration-dependent relaxation in arterial segments pre-stimulated with phenylephrine (1 μM). The relaxations evoked by both agents were closely related to repolarisation of the smooth muscle cell membrane potential. However, in the presence of raised extracellular potassium repolarisation to SIN-1 was inhibited to a much greater extent than relaxation. In contrast, the attenuation of acetylcholine-evoked relaxation observed in the presence of raised potassium was mirrored by reduced repolarisation. Exposure to 1H-[1,2,4]oxadiazolo[4,3-a]quinoxalin-1-one (ODQ; 10 μM) almost completely inhibited both relaxation and repolarisation to SIN-1 but only reduced relaxation and repolarisation to acetylcholine and to exogenous nitric oxide by 40 %.

These data indicate that different mechanisms underlie arterial relaxation to the nitric oxide donor SIN-1, endothelium-derived and authentic nitric oxide. SIN-1-evoked relaxation and repolarisation both appear to be mediated by activation of soluble guanylyl cyclase. In contrast, relaxation to endothelium-derived and exogenous nitric oxide are largely independent of cyclic GMP and may be mediated by direct activation of potassium channels leading to smooth muscle repolarisation.

Supported by the Wellcome Trust (UK).

111

PULSATILE STRETCH ENSURES THE CONTINUOUS RELEASE OF ENDOTHELIUM-DERIVED HYPERPOLARIZING FACTOR IN PORCINE CORONARY ARTERIES.

R. Popp, I. Fleming, J. Bauersachs, R. Busse.
Institut für Kardiovaskuläre Physiologie, Klinikum der J.W.Goethe-Universität, Theodor-Stern-Kai 7, 60590 Frankfurt am Main, Germany.

The endothelium-derived hyperpolarizing factor, which may be a cytochrome P450-derived metabolite of arachidonic acid, hyperpolarises underlying vascular smooth muscle cells by activating Ca^{2+} dependent K^+ channels. We investigated whether the release of EDHF could also be elicited in response to rhythmic deformation of porcine coronary arteries. Arterial segments, pre-incubated with N^Gnitro-L-arginine and diclofenac, were cannulated and exposed to pulsatile changes in intraluminal pressure (1 Hz, 2 min, 30 to 90 mmHg) the EDHF-containing perfusate was withdrawn and applied to detector rat aortic smooth muscle cells, the membrane potential of which was continuously measured using the patch-clamp technique. The EDHF-induced hyperpolarization of detector cells was proportional to the amplitude of the pulsatile change in pressure applied to the donor artery: control, 0 mV; 30 mmHg, -1.6±0.1 mV; 60 mmHg, -3.3±0.2 mV and 90 mmHg, -6.6±0.4 mV. Pulsatile pressure failed to elicit the release of a hyperpolarising factor from endothelium-denuded segments. Pre-incubation of endothelium-intact donor arteries with 17-octadecynoic acid (3 µM), a specific cytochrome P450 inhibitor markedly attenuated the pulsatile pressure-induced release of EDHF, as assessed by the hyperpolarization of detector cells (hyperpolarization was decreased from -5.5 to -1.5 mV). The simultaneous application of EDHF-containing perfusate and either tetrabutylammonium (3 mM) or iberiotoxin (10 nM), two inhibitors of Ca^{2+} sensitive K^+ channels significantly reduced the subsequent hyperpolarization of detector smooth muscle cells. These findings demonstrate for the first time that the synthesis of EDHF can be mechanically stimulated by rhythmic vessel wall distention, and suggest that EDHF may be continuously released and contribute to the control of coronary blood flow.

112

PHENYLEPHRINE ENHANCES RELAXATION BY $BETA_1$- BUT NOT $BETA_2$-AGONISTS IN PULMONARY ARTERIES

R. M. Priest, D. Hucks, J. P. T. Ward
Department of Allergy and Respiratory Medicine, UMDS St Thomas' Campus, London SE1 7EH, U.K.

In pulmonary arteries constricted with prostaglandin $F_{2\alpha}$ the large majority of ß-adrenoceptor-induced relaxation is mediated by nitric oxide. We show here that relationship is altered following constriction with the α-agonist phenylephrine. Arteries were mounted on a myograph and contracted with either 10µM phenylephrine or 50µM prostaglandin $F_{2\alpha}$, to give approximately equivalent tensions. Concentration-response curves were obtained for isoprenaline, salbutamol and forskolin, and following inhibition of nitric oxide synthesis with 100µM L-NMMA. Isoprenaline has some α-agonist activity in this preparation, and experiments with prostaglandin $F_{2\alpha}$ were performed in the presence of 10µM phentolamine. Results are mean ± S.E.M.

Isoprenaline caused a much greater maximum relaxation in arteries constricted with phenylephrine (87±7%, n=6) than those with prostaglandin $F_{2\alpha}$ (38±4%, n=6, p<0.01). The difference was not significant for salbutamol (PE: 49±8%, n=6; $PGF_{2\alpha}$: 35±7%, n=6, NS). L-NMMA greatly reduced maximum relaxation to isoprenaline in arteries constricted with prostaglandin $F_{2\alpha}$ (5±1%, n=4), but only reduced relaxation by 50% in those constricted by phenylephrine (43±4%, n=5). L-NMMA substantially reduced relaxation to salbutamol for both vasoconstrictors (PE: 9±3, n=5; $PGF_{2\alpha}$: 8±1%, n=4; NS). The EC_{50} for forskolin was shifted to the left in arteries constricted with phenylephrine (PE: 41±7nM, n=6; $PGF_{2\alpha}$: 267±28nM, n=6; p<0.01). These results suggest that in this tissue there is functional cross-talk between α- and $ß_1$-, but not $ß_2$-, adrenoceptor pathways, which may involve cAMP. Supported by the British Heart Foundation.

113

CALCIUM-TENSION RELATIONSHIP DURING CONTRACTION INDUCED BY EXO- AND ENDOGENOUSLY APPLIED NOR-ADRENALINE IN RAT MESENTERIC RESISTANCE ARTERIES

N.J.H. Raat, G.E.C. Wetzels, and J.G.R. De Mey.
Department of Pharmacology, Universiteit Maastricht, P.O.Box 616, 6200 MD, Maastricht, The Netherlands.

Calcium-tension relationships were constructed in isolated rat mesenteric resistance arteries (n=8) that had been mounted for the recording of isometric force development and loaded with Fura-2/AM. Before experiments, sensory motor nerves were depleted of neuropeptides and 1 µM of each nitro-L-arginine, indomethacin, and propranolol were present throughout the experiment. First, it was shown that noradrenaline (NA, 10 µM) induced an additional increase in tension without a further change in intracellular calcium concentration ($[Ca^{2+}]_i$) during incubation with 125 mM K^+. Subsequently, cumulative concentration-response curves were constructed for NA (0.6 to 10 µM), electrical field stimulation of sympathetic nerves (EFS, 1 to 16 Hz) and for 5.9 to 125 mM K^+ before and after exposure to the irreversible α-adrenoceptor blocker phenoxybenzamine (POB). Calcium-tension relationships obtained during NA, EFS and K^+ were shifted to the left of those observed during K^+ after POB. After treatment with POB, $[Ca^{2+}]_i$ was increased at a given extracellular K^+ concentration and tension was reduced at a given $[Ca^{2+}]_i$. In conclusion, these results confirm that stimulation of α-adrenoceptors increases the sensitivity of the arterial smooth muscle contractile apparatus for calcium. In addition, it was shown that this not only applies for exogenously supplied noradrenaline, but also for endogenously released noradrenaline from nerve endings. Moreover, these results suggest that the observed calcium-sensitization is accompanied by a reduction of the intracellular calcium level.

114

ROLE OF NITRIC OXIDE FOR SKELETAL MUSCLE BLOOD FLOW REGULATION

G. Rådegran, and B. Saltin.
CMRC, Rigshospitalet, Tagensvej 20, DK-2200, Copenhagen, Denmark.

NO is postulated to regulate basal vascular tone in skeletal muscle of man at rest. Different isoforms of NO synthase has in relation to skeletal muscle been localized to the sarcolemma, mitochondria, and vascular endothelium - suggesting a role for NO in linking delivery and substrate utilization to the elevated local metabolic demand during exercise. Our objective was to determine the role of NO for exercise hyperemia.

Blood flow was measured with Ultrasound Doppler in the femoral artery of six healthy male subjects at rest, during, and in recovery from one-legged dynamic knee extensor exercise - prior to and during NOS blockade by infusion of L-NMMA in the femoral artery (5 $mg*min^{-1}*l^{-1}$ for 5 min, thereafter 1 $mg*min^{-1}*l^{-1}$ thigh volume). NOS blockade at rest decreased blood flow by 55% from 0.39 ±0.08 $l*min^{-1}$, increased mean arterial pressure with 8 ±2 mmHg, whereas leg oxygen uptake (22 ±4 $ml*min^{-1}$) and heart rate (53 ±3 min^{-1}) was unaltered. The blockade did neither effect the initial rate of rise or the magnitude of blood flow (4.82 ±0.4 $l*min^{-1}$), mean arterial pressure (122 ±3 mmHg), heart rate (98 ±5 min^{-1}), and leg oxygen uptake at 70% of work rate max, nor the blood flow (7.60 ±1.04 $l*min^{-1}$), mean arterial pressure (148 ±8 mmHg), or leg oxygen uptake at termination of peak exercise, whereas peak heart rate of 137 ±3 min^{-1} was lowered by 10%. Recovery blood flow was reduced by 46%, whereas the leg oxygen uptake was similar. In conclusion, our data confirms the role of NO for regulating skeletal muscle blood flow at rest, and during recovery, but neither at onset of, steady state, or peak dynamic exercise.

115

EFFECTS OF DIETARY L-ARGININE ON REACTIVITY OF CANINE CORONARY ARTERIES

E. C. Ray, M. E. Landis and V. M. Miller
Departments of Surgery and Physiology and Biophysics, Mayo Graduate School of Medicine, Mayo Foundation, Rochester, MN. USA

Experiments were designed to determine effects of dietary supplementation with L-arginine on endothelial function of canine coronary arteries. Left circumflex coronary arteries were removed from two groups of dogs four weeks after bilateral reversed saphenous vein grafts were interposed into femoral arteries. One group of dogs received oral L-arginine supplementation (200mg/kg/day). All dogs received aspirin (325mg/day). Rings cut from coronary arteries were suspended for the measurement of isometric force in organ chambers. In the presence of indomethacin (10^{-5}M), concentration-response curves to L-arginine (10^{-8} to 10^{-3}M) were obtained the in absence and presence of either N^G-monomethyl-L-arginine (L-NMMA; 10^{-4}M) or tetraethylammonium (TEA; 10^{-3}M) during contractions to prostaglandin $F_{2\alpha}$. Steady-state serum concentrations of L-arginine increased by 10% with L-arginine feeding. In coronary arteries from control dogs, L-arginine caused endothelium and concentration-dependent contractions which were reduced by either L-NMMA or TEA. On the contrary, in arteries from arginine-fed dogs, L-arginine caused endothelium, concentration-dependent contractions only in the presence of TEA. These results suggest L-arginine can alter contractions of canine coronary arteries by at least two mechanisms in endothelial cells: activation of potassium channels and production of nitric oxide. When circulating concentrations of L-arginine are increased by dietary supplementation, the relative contribution of each of these mechanisms is altered.

116

EFFECT OF HYPERCHOLESTEROLEMIA ON NITRIC OXIDE AND ENDOTHELIUM-DERIVED HYPERPOLARIZING FACTOR MEDIATED VASORELAXATION IN PORCINE CORONARY ARTERIES

A.D. Freay, T. Portelle, M. Werner, P. Verhallen, G.M. Rubanyi
Department of Cardiovascular Research, Berlex Biosciences, Richmond, CA 94804, USA

Endothelium-dependent relaxation to bradykinin is mediated by both nitric oxide (NO) and endothelium-derived hyperpolarizing factor (EDHF) in porcine coronary arteries [Kauser and Rubanyi. J Cardiovasc Pharmac 1992; 20: S101-104]. The present study was designed to test for the first time the effect of high lipid feeding on NO and EDHF production in coronary arteries with intact endothelium isolated from male Yucatan minipigs. In order to separate NO- and EDHF-mediated responses, bradykinin-induced relaxations were tested in the presence of ibuprofen ($3x10^{-6}$ M) under the following conditions: 1) contraction with the thromboxane analogue, U46619 (10^{-8} M) (combined NO- and EDHF-mediated relaxation), 2) U46619 and N^G-nitro-L-arginine (LNNA; 10^{-4} M) (EDHF-mediated relaxation), and 3) contraction with KC1 (40mM) (NO-mediated relaxation) (Kauser and Rubanyi; 1992). High lipid feeding of castrated animals for 4 and 8 weeks caused progressive suppression of EDHF- but not of NO-mediated endothelium-dependent vasorelaxation. In conclusion, these studies show that short-term hypercholesterolemia selectively impairs EDHF-mediated endothelium dependent relaxation in porcine coronary arteries.

117

LONG-LASTING PRODUCTION OF CYCLIC GMP BY CULTURED SMOOTH MUSCLE CELLS FROM ATHEROSCLEROTIC RABBIT AORTA.

A. Rupin, D. Behr, F. Jaunault, T. J. Verbeuren.
Division of Angiology, Servier Research Institute, 92150 Suresnes, France.

Evidence for a functional non-endothelial NO-synthase associated with an increased cyclase GMP production has been reported in aortas of hypercholesterolemic rabbits (Verbeuren TJ et al., J. Cardiovasc. Pharmacol., 1993 ; 21 : 841-845 ; Rupin A et al., Brit. J. Pharmacol., 1996 ; 119 : 1233-1258).

To study the activity of soluble guanylate cyclase in viable non-broken smooth muscle cells from atherosclerotic rabbit aortas, smooth muscle cells were cultured from aortic medial explants from New-Zealand white rabbits fed a control diet or a 0.3 % cholesterol diet for 45 weeks. Intracellular a well as extracellular cyclic GMP levels in response to interleukin-1β and sodium nitroprusside were measured. Intracellular cyclic GMP levels were not modified in response to interleukin 1β at 100 UI/ml and were increased after 3, 6 and 24 hours of incubation with 100 μM of sodium nitroprusside. In contrast, extracellular cyclic GMP production was increased between 6 and 24 hours with atherosclerotic smooth muscle cells in comparison to control cells for both stimuli.

This study demonstrates a long lasting production of cyclic GMP in response to NO in cultured smooth muscle cells from atherosclerotic rabbit aorta and provides evidence for increased activity of guanylate cyclase in atherosclerotic smooth muscle cells.

118

AMELIORATION OF CORONARY MICROVASCULOPATHY AND ENDOTHELIUM-DEPENDENT RELAXATION IN DIABETIC RATS BY AN INHIBITOR OF PLASMINOGEN ACTIVATOR, IRSOGLADIN

I. Sakuma, Y. Hattori*, M. Gao**, T. Koyama**, A. Sato, A. Tamada, Y. Akaishi, D. Goto, T. Tomioka, S. Fujii, M. Fukao*, M. Kanno*, A. Kitabatake
Departments of Cardiovascular Medicine and *Pharmacology, School of Medicine, and **Research Institute of Electric Science, Hokkaido University, Sapporo 060, Japan

Pathogenesis of microvasculopathy and the impairment of endothelium-dependent relaxation in type I diabetes mellitus are attributed to hyperglycemia. We have previously shown that insulin treatment of streptozotocin-treated rats increases plasminogen activator inhibitor-1 immunostaining in coronary microvessels in vivo. To determine whether hyperfibrinolysis due to low plasminogen activator inhibitor-1 in insulin deficient diabetes plays a direct role in microvasculopathy and impaired coronary function we examined the effects of irsogladin, a potent inhibitor of plasminogen activator, which is clinically used to treat peptic ulcer.

Single streptozotocin treatment (45 mg/kg, i.v.) rendered male Wistar rats diabetic and dystrophic. Insulin (6 IU/day, s.c.), but not irsogladin (4 mg/day, p.o.), prevented hyperglycemia and dystrophy. After 3 months coronary microvessels of the diabetic rats exhibited markedly increased tortuosity, and bradykinin-induced coronary relaxation of perfused isolated heart in the presence or absence of L-N^G-nitroarginine was impaired. Both insulin and irsogladin prevented the microvasculopathy and irsogladin ameliorated the bradykinin-induced coronary relaxation.

Thus, insulin deficiency and subsequent hyperfibrinolysis due to low plasminogen activator inhibitor-1 expression may impair integrity of coronary microvessels and the endothelium-dependent relaxation.

119

INFLUENCE OF NITRIC OXIDE RELEASE ON THE CONTRACTILE RESPONSE TO SEROTONIN OF BASILAR ARTERY FROM WISTAR KYOTO AND STROKE-PRONE RATS

S. Salomone, N. Morel, T. Godfraind
Laboratoire de Pharmacologie, Université Catholique de Louvain, Avenue Hippocrate 54, UCL 5410, B-1200 Brussels, Belgium.

In this study we examined if differences in nitric oxide release could contribute to the difference in sensitivity to serotonin of basilar arteries from Wistar Kyoto and stroke-prone rats. Isolated basilar arteries were studied in wire myograph.

The relaxing effect of acetylcholine (3 µM) added on the contraction to serotonin (1 µM) was higher in Wistar Kyoto rats than in stroke-prone rats ($P<0.01$). The potency of serotonin was higher in in stroke-prone than in Wistar Kyoto arteries ($P<0.01$). Rubbing of endothelium produced a shift to the left of the serotonin curve in Wistar Kyoto ($P<0.01$), but not in stroke-prone arteries. N^{ω}-nitro-L-arginine (0.1 mM) produced a similar increase in tone in both Wistar Kyoto and stroke-prone arteries, equal to about 70% of 100 mM KCl-evoked contraction, this tone was absent when the arteries were bathed in phosphate-free Krebs. In such medium, the blockade of NO synthase increased the potency of serotonin in Wistar Kyoto ($P<0.01$), but not in stroke-prone arteries.

These results show that endothelium-dependent vasorelaxation to acetylcholine is impaired in stroke-prone arteries. The finding that removal of endothelium or blockade of NO synthase augmented the contractile response to serotonin in Wistar Kyoto, but not in stroke-prone basilar arteries indicates that the difference in responsiveness to serotonin observed between basilar arteries might be, at least in part, related to dissimilarities in NO release.

120

ENDOTHELIAL DYSFUNCTION BY GLYCOSYLATED HUMAN OXYHEMOGLOBIN DEPENDS ON THE OXYDATIVE STATE OF THE HEME GROUP

C. F. Sánchez-Ferrer, J. Angulo, C. Peiró, A. Sánchez-Ferrer, P. López-Dóriga, L. Rodríguez-Mañas
Departamento de Farmacología y Terapéutica, Facultad de Medicina, Universidad Autónoma de Madrid, and Unidad de Investigación y Servicio de Geriatría, Hospital Universitario de Getafe, Madrid, Spain

Nanomolar highly glycosylated oxyhemoglobin impairs endothelial function by releasing superoxide anions (Angulo J et Al. Hypertension 1996; 28: 583-592). Whether these effects are linked to the oxidative state of the hemoglobin or they are non-specific, i.e. they can be observed with other circulating glycosylated proteins, is not known. We analyzed if the endothelial dysfunction induced by glycosylated hemoglobin is present when the iron atoms are oxydized to ferric trivalent state, by testing the influence of 14%-glycosylated human methemoglobin and cyanomethemoglobin on endothelium-dependent relaxations induced by acetylcholine (10 nM to 10 µM) in isolated aortic rings from non-diabetic Sprague-Dawley rats. To check another circulating protein, 14%-glycosylated bovine seroalbumin was also tested. At physiological (nanomolar) concentrations, only 14%-glycosylated oxyhemoglobin caused contractile responses or the impairment of endothelium-dependent relaxations. These effects were inhibited by 100 U/ml superoxide dismutase. Both met- and cyanomethemoglobin, either non glycosylated or 14%-glycosylated, did not alter endothelial function. Similar lack of effects were observed with non-glycosylated and glycosylated bovine seroalbumin (up to 300 µM). Therefore, the present results suggest that the endothelial dysfunction produced by nanomolar glycosylated hemoglobin is due to superoxide anion production and requires a functional heme group containing iron in ferrous state. It seems unlikely that albumin glycosylation could have a role on determining endothelial impairment.

121

EFFECTS OF LOCAL WARMING, SODIUM NITROPRUSSIDE AND BRETYLIUM IONTOPHORESIS ON CUTANEOUS VASODILATION OF THE HAND

J.L. Saumet, M. Saumet, G. Leftheriotis, P Abraham, A Jardel.
Laboratoire de physiologie, C.H.U. 49033 Angers cedex 01, France

Local warming to 42°C induces a greater cutaneous vasodilation than reactive hyperhemia following 10 min. of ischemia. This vasodilation has been considered as maximal and its value to be characteristic of each individual. However, we do not know if the blockade of the release of transmitter from the adrenergic nerve endings or a direct pharmacological action on vascular smooth muscle by a vasodilator substance can increase skin blood flow more than local warming.

We performed three experiments in which skin blood flow was measured by Laser Doppler flowmetry on the dorsal aspect of the hand. Twelve healthy subjects participated in the experimental trials. Each experiment began by a 3 min. period of ischemia and its subsequent reactive hyperemia. The vasodilator effect of 20 min. of local warming at 44°C ($n=14$); iontophoresis of sodium nitroprusside ($n=11$) and iontophoresis of bretylium tosylate ($n=10$) were measured: mean+/-SEM. Skin blood flow increased from 24.0+/-5.7 to 64.9+/-10.4 A.U. ($p<0.01$), from 30.2+/-7.9 to 128.1+/-16.2 A.U. ($p<0.01$) and from 24.4+/-2.5 to 151.0+/-15.0 A.U. ($p<0.001$) during local warming, sodium nitroprusside and bretylium iontophoresis respectively.

We conclude that the effects of iontophoresis of sodium nitroprusside or bretylium produce a cutaneous vasodilation higher than a local warming on the dorsal aspect of the hand. Therefore, local warming does not induce a maximal vasodilation of skin capillaries on the human hand.

122

INFLUENCE OF TOPICAL CAPSAICIN ON LOCAL THERMAL CONTROL OF THE HUMAN CUTANEOUS CIRCULATION

J.L. Saumet, D.P. Stephens, N. Charkoudian, J. Mueller, J.M. Johnson.
Laboratoire de physiologie et d'explorations vasculaires, Centre hosp. Universitaire, 49033 Angers cedex 01 France and Dept. Physiology Univ. Texas health Sci. Ctr. San Antonio TX 78284 USA.

Topical capsaicin treatment acutely raises skin blod flow and excites warm receptors, similar to direct warming. We studied the effects of capsaicin on the relationship of skin blood flow to local temperature and warm receptor activity. Part 1: effects of capsaicin on the forearm skin blood flow-local temperature relationship were assessed by laser Doppler flowmetry 1 hour after topical capsaicin (0.075%). The area was cooled to 29°C and rewarmed stepwise to 42°C. Vasodilation and heat sensation began at a local temperature 6.03+/-0.81°C lower than at untreated sites ($p<0.05$), shifting the blood flow-local temperature relationship to the right. A smaller shift (3.12+/-0.72°C) occured with lower concentration capsaicin cream (0.025%). Part 2: A site treated with 0.025% capsaicin was cooled below the threshold for warmth perception and rewarmed in 1-2°C steps. At each step, an untreated site on the opposite arm was warmed until the subject perceived the temperature to be the same as at the treated site. This design provided similar warm receptor activation at different temeratures. At treated sites, skin blood flow was higher relative to actual temperature ($p<0.05$). However, there was not a significant difference between sites in the relationship of blood flow to perceived temperature, presumably reflecting similar warm receptor activity. These findings suggest a role for warm receptor activation in the vasodilator response to local warming.

123

EX VIVO TRANSFECTION OF TYPE III NITRIC OXIDE SYNTHASE INTO CANINE SAPHENOUS VEINS

S. R. Severson, C. G. A. McGregor and V. M. Miller
Departments of Surgery and Physiology and Biophysics, Mayo Clinic and Foundation, Rochester, MN, USA

Experiments were designed to characterize function of canine saphenous veins after liposome mediated transfection of the recombinant gene for Type III nitric oxide synthase (endothelial, ecNOS). Under sterile conditions, canine saphenous veins were perfused under pressure (90 mm Hg, one hour) with a liposome:plasmid (1:1) complex (10 μg liposomal complex/ml of Medium) with and without (control) the gene construct for ecNOS. Following incubation for 24 hours at 37°C, transfection was verified using polymerase chain reaction (PCR); no transfected gene was detected in control veins. Calcium-dependent activity of isolated nitric oxide synthase was greater in ecNOS-transfected compared to control veins. However, accumulation of oxidized products of nitric oxide (NO_x) measured in the incubation media of rings of veins stimulated with acetylcholine ($3x10^{-7}M$) was the same in media from ecNOS-transfected and control veins. Results indicate the feasibility of using *ex vivo* liposomal transfection for gene delivery to veins. The transfection procedure resulted in increased activity of the enzyme product of the transfected gene. However, expression of enzyme activity in tissue may be modulated or limited by availability of co-factors, substrate or interaction of the enzyme with intracellular reactive oxygen species.

124

ESCAPE FROM PRESSOR ACTION OF ANGIOTENSIN-2: ROLE OF NITRIC OXIDE

V.I.Shebeko
Department of Pathophysiology, Vitebsk Medical Institute, Vitebsk 210023, Belarus

It is well known that intravenous infusion of angiotensin-2 causes at first a rise in the mean arterial pressure, but then it falls, inspite of the continued infusion of angiotensin-2, i.e. a phenomenon of "escape" from the pressor action of angiotensin-2 is seen. The aim of the experiments was to study the role of nitric oxide in the development of this phenomenon of "escape".

The experiments were carried out on female-rats anesthetized with nembuthal. The following mixtures were injected intravenously for a period of 10 minutes: (1) angiotensin-2 (0,5 mcg/kg/min); (2) angiotensin-2 + L-NG-Monomethylarginine (1,25 mg/kg/min); (3) angiotensin-2 + L-NG-Monomethylarginine + L-arginine (3,0 mg/kg/min). At the 10-th minute of infusion the degree of "escape" was determined as percent of the fall in mean arterial pressure from its maximim rise.

Under conditions of normal formation of nitric oxide, the degree of "escape" was 60,9 $\pm$ 5,8 %. The NO-synthase inhibitor eliminated the "escape" phenomenon (the degree of "escape" was 1,8 $\pm$ 1,0 %) and L-arginine restored the "escape" again (the degree of "escape" was 39,5 $\pm$ 4,4 %).

This data shows that this phenomenon of "escape" from the pressor action of angiotensin-2 is related to an increased production of nitric oxide.

125

ROLE OF NITRIC OXIDE IN COMPLEMENT-INDUCED ARTERIAL HYPOTENSION

V.I. Shebeko
Department of Pathophysiology, Vitebsk Medical Institute, Vitebsk 210023, Byelorussia

The aim of the experiments was to determine the role of nitric oxide in the development of arterial hypotension during the complement activation.

The experiments were carried out on female-rats anesthetized with nembuthal. A model of intravascular activation of the complement was created by repeated intravenous injections of zymosan. We studied (1) the effect of the inhibition of NO-synthase on the degree of arterial hypotension; (2) the contractile response of the aortal ring to noradrenaline and serotonin.

A preliminary intravenous injection of L-NG-Monomethylarginine markedly reduces the degree of acute arterial hypotension during the intravascular complement activation. Intravenous injection of NO-synthase inhibitor caused a larger increase in mean arterial pressure after the activation of the complement than in the control group. After a 2-hour complement activation, the contractile response of the aortal ring to the action of noradrenaline and serotonin decreased. The NO-synthase inhibitor restored the contractile response of the aorta to these agents.

In conclusion, an increase in the formation of nitric oxide can take part in the development of arterial hypotension during the intravascular complement activation.

126

HIGH DENSITY LIPOPROTEIN INDUCES VASORELAXATION AND VASOCONSTRICTION OF PORCINE CORONARY ARTERY

Issei Shimada, Takao Okada, Hiroshi Yamaguchi*, Rikuo Ochi
Depts. of Physiology and Cardiology*, Juntendo Univ. Sch. of Med. Hongo 2-1-1, Bunkyo-ku, Tokyo 113, Japan

The amount of high density lipoprotein (HDL) inversely correlates with the incidence of atherosclerotic diseases. However, little is known of the effects of HDL on vasculer tonus. We examined acute effects of native HDL on the isolated strips of porcine right coronary artery. HDL was obtained by ultracentrifuging collected from human plasma from healthy normolipemic volunteers. The isolated coronary strips (2x10mm), were vertically mounted in organ chambers and were precontracted with prostaglandin (PG) F2α (6μM). Application of HDL (500μg protein/ml) on endothelium intact arteries induced evident vasorelaxation (n=11); isometrical tension developed by PGF2α was significantly ($p<0.05$) diminished by HDL by -12.8 ± 1.4% of the maximal tension at 20min. N^G-monomethyl-L-arginine (300μM), a nitric oxide synthase inhibitor, did not affect the HDL-induced vasorelaxation while AA861 (10μM), a lipoxygenase inhibitor augmented the HDL-induced vasorelaxation (-28.2±3.6% at 20min, n=5). On the other hand, pretreatment by indomethacin (10μM), a cyclooxygenase inhibitor, reversed the HDL-induced vasorelaxation to vasoconstriction (vasoconstriction by 10.4±2.1% of the PGF2α-induced maximal tension at 20min, n=6). In endothelium denuded strips (n=4), HDL exerted neither vasorelaxing nor vasoconstriction effect. These results indicate that HDL is capable to cause vasorelaxation via, at least in part, endothelium derived cyclooxygenase (COX) product(s) such as PGI_2 and also to cause vasoconstriction through lipoxygenase pathway possibly by leucotriene when COX activity is lowered.

127

THE ROLE OF INFLAMMATORY CYTOKINES IN THE PATHOGENESIS OF CORONARY ARTERIOSCLEROSIS AND VASOSPASTIC RESPONSES IN PIGS IN VIVO

H. Shimokawa
Research Institute of Angiocardiology and Cardiovascular Clinic, Kyushu University School of Medicine, Fukuoka 812-82, Japan.

Studies in vitro have suggested that inflammatory cytokines may play an important role in the pathogenesis of arteriosclerosis. However, little is known about their effects in vivo. The present study was thus designed to determine their role in coronary arteriosclerosis in pigs in vivo.

Under aseptic conditions, proximal segments of the left porcine coronary arteries were gently wrapped with cotton mesh absorbing sepharose beads with or without recombinant human interleukin-1β (or other cytokines). From 1 to 4 weeks after the operation, coronary intimal lesions and vasospastic responses to intracoronary serotonin or histamine were induced at the cytokine-treated site but not at the control site. Those histological and functional changes induced by the chronic treatment with interleukin-1β were significantly inhibited by the simultaneous treatment with a neutralizing antibody either to interleukin-1β, platelet-derived growth factor or basic fibroblast growth factor. Furthermore, interleukin-1β-induced coronary changes were markedly suppressed by co-treatment with ST 638, a specific tyrosine kinase inhibitor.

These results indicate that (1) inflammatory cytokines play an important role in the pathogenesis of coronary arteriosclerosis and vasospatic responses in vivo and (2) growth factors are substantially involved in the cytokine-induced coronary inflammatory/proliferative changes via activation of tyrosine kinases in vivo.

128

CAPILLARY PRESSURE IN ACUTE HYPOXAEMIA

D.M. Lewis,*+ A.R. Bradwell,*^ S. Watts,*" A.C. Shore+
^Birmingham Med Res Expeditionary Soc, "Dept Environmental & Occupational Med, Aberdeen Univ.+Inst Clin Sci, PGMS, Exeter Univ.

Rapid exposure to high altitude may result in peripheral oedema, proteinuria and potentially cerebral and pulmonary oedema. The microvascular basis of the oedema formation is unclear. This study, which was approved by the Medical Research Ethics Committee, investigated the effects of acute hypoxia on capillary pressure

Eight subjects (28-56 years 3F) were studied at <200m above sea level and after overnight exposure to a simulated altitude of 4000m in a hypobaric chamber. All subjects gave written informed consent and all had experience at high altitude. Capillary pressure was measured by direct cannulation of the apex of several finger nailfold capillaries by glass micropipette using a servonulling feedback system. Dorsal hand vein pressure was measured by indwelling cannula. Ambient temperature was equal for baseline and altitude studies. Subjects had varying degrees of acute mountain sickness, Lake Louise scores 8 (4-13) median (range), scores of ≥ 3 indicating acute mountain sickness. The partial pressure of oxygen measured in arterialised ear lobe capillary blood gas was 5.03 (4.62-5.9) kPa after altitude exposure. Capillary pressure rose from 14.5 (9.0-18.1) mmHg to 16.7 (12.1-18.3) mmHg $p<0.05$, Wilcoxon signed rank test. There was no correlation between capillary pressure and acute mountain sickness scores. Venous pressure rose from 8.4 (7.9-12.5) mmHg to 11.9 (8.0-17.2), $p<0.05$.

Acute mountain sickness is clearly multifactorial: We have previously shown an increase in hydraulic conductance (Lewis DM et al. Eur J Clin Invest 1997 (in press)) and have now demonstrated a rise in capillary pressure, which may contribute to the formation of oedema.

129

MECHANISMS UNDERLYING ESTROGEN INHIBITION OF $[Ca^{2+}]i$ IN CORONARY ARTERY SMOOTH MUSCLE.

G.C. Sieck, Y.S. Prakash, M.S. Kannan, and V.M. Miller.
Mayo Foundation, Rochester, MN, USA.

Experiments were designed to study the mechanisms by which 17β-estradiol (17β-E_2) inhibits intracellular Ca^{2+} ($[Ca^{2+}]i$) in acutely dissociated porcine coronary artery smooth muscle (CSM) cells. In response to 100nM endothelin-1, $[Ca^{2+}]i$ increased from ~100 nM to ~ 600 nM. In gonadally-intact, sexually mature female pigs, where the presence of estrogen receptors in CSM cells was confirmed by receptor binding assay, 17β-E_2 inhibited the endothelin-1 induced elevation in $[Ca^{2+}]i$ in a concentration-dependent (0.1 nM to 100 nM) fashion. This inhibitory effect of 17β-E_2 was blocked by the specific estrogen receptor antagonist ICI 182,780 (IC_{50} 10nM). In addition, the inhibition of the endothelin-1 induced $[Ca^{2+}]i$ response was not observed in CSM cells from ovariectomized pigs, where the absence of estrogen receptors was confirmed. In CSM cells from intact pigs, 17β-E_2 also blocked the elevation of $[Ca^{2+}]i$ induced by BayK8644, indicating an inhibition of Ca^{2+} influx through voltage-gated channels. When both Ca^{2+} influx (zero extracellular Ca^{2+} and/or nifedipine) and SR Ca^{2+} reuptake (by thapsigargin) were blocked, $[Ca^{2+}]i$ gradually increased. Under this condition, 17β-E_2 caused a reduction in $[Ca^{2+}]i$, indicating an enhancement of Ca^{2+} efflux. However, when both Ca^{2+} influx and efflux were blocked by zero extracellular Ca^{2+} and lanthanum, 17β-E_2 did not affect SR Ca^{2+} release induced either by endothelin-1 or caffeine. Together, these data indicate that, in addition to inhibiting Ca^{2+} influx, 17β-E_2 also increases Ca^{2+} efflux, thereby decreasing $[Ca^{2+}]i$.

130

EFFECTS OF SOLUBLE GUANYLATE CYCLASE INHIBITION CONFIRM NON-ENDOTHELIAL NITRIC OXIDE SYNTHASE ACTIVITY IN ATHEROSCLEROTIC RABBIT AORTA.

S. Simonet, E. Bonhomme, G. Lavielle and T.J. Verbeuren.
Division of Angiology, Servier Research Institute, 92150 Suresnes, France.

Nitric oxide (NO) derived from non-endothelial inducible NO-synthase is probably at the origin of reduced contractions to alpha-adrenoceptor agonists in atherosclerotic aortas (Verbeuren TJ et al. J Cardiovasc Pharmacol 1993; 21:841-845). The aim of the present study was to confirm the inducible NO-synthase activity in atherosclerosis using a selective inhibitor of the soluble guanylate cyclase, 1H-[1,2,4] oxadiazolo [4,3,-a] quinoxalin-1-one (ODQ). Rings with and without endothelium of aortas from control or cholesterol-fed (30 weeks; 0.3 %) rabbits were mounted for isometric tension recording.

In control aortas, the NO-synthase inhibitor, nitro-L-arginine (1-100 μM) and ODQ (0.1-10 μM) dose-dependently augmented the contractions to phenylephrine in rings with but not in those without endothelium; ODQ (10 μM) inhibited nitroglycerin- and acetylcholine-induced relaxations, but not those caused by CNP-22. In contrast, both nitro-L-arginine and ODQ dose-dependently augmented the contractions to phenylephrine in atherosclerotic aortas with and without endothelium; the nitro-L-arginine-induced effects were reversed by L-arginine (1 mM) and those of ODQ were completely inhibited by nitro-L-arginine(100 μM). In the atherosclerotic aortas, ODQ inhibited the nitroglycerin-induced relaxations.

These data confirm the activity of an inducible non-endothelial NO-synthase in the atherosclerotic rabbit aorta. They are in agreement with augmented cGMP production recently reported in this tissue (Rupin A et al. Brit J Pharmacol 1996;119:1233-1238).

131

INVOLVEMENT OF ENDOTHELIUM ON THE ANTI-HYPERTENSIVE EFFECT OF CLONIDINE

R. Soares de Moura & M. Cardoso Leão
Depart. Farmacologia, Univ. Estado do Rio de Janeiro. Av 28 de Setembro, 87 - CEP 20 551-090 Rio de Janeiro Brasil

The mechanism of the anti-hypertensive effect of clonidine is not completely elucidate but it is probably due to reduction of symphatetic tone mediated by stimulation of central α_2 adrenoceptors. As activation of α_2-adrenoceptors on the endothelial cells induces release of EDRF, we decide to find out if activation of endothelium α_2-adrenoceptors is involved on the anti-hypertensive action of clonidine. Therefore the hypotensive effect of clonidine was studied in control and in L-NAME or methylene blue treated rats. Wistar rats (280-380g) were anaesthetized with chloralose (130mg/kg ip). Systolic and diastolic arterial blood pressure were recorded on a Hewlett Packard polygraph. Intravenous injection of clonidine (10 μg/kg n=8, control group) caused a rapid increase of arterial blood pressure (Δ increase of 63.2±5.2 and 36.8±1.9 mm Hg for systolic and diastolic blood pressure respectively), followed by a long lasting hypotensive effect (Δ decrease of diastolic blood pressure 53.0±4.6 mm Hg, 20 minutes after injection). The hypotensive effect estimated as AUC during 20 minutes was 598.5±100. Clonidine (10μ/kg n=5) injected 10 minutes after pretreatment with L-NAME (10mg/kg iv) did not induce decrease in arterial blood pressure. Clonidine (10μg/kg iv, n=9) injected 5 minutes after methylene blue (10mg/kg iv) induced a hypotensive effect (AUC 265.73) that was significantly smaller than control group (P<0.03). These results suggest that nitric oxide released by activation of α_2-adrenoceptors may play a very important role on the mechanism of the anti-hypertensive effect of clonidine.

132

AUTOREGULATION OF CORONARY FLOW IN ISOLATED RAT'S HEART AFTER BLOCADE OF NITRIC OXIDE PRODUCTION

A.P. Solodkov
Department of Normal Physiology, Medical Institute, Vitebsk, 210023, Belarus.

On isolated Langendorff rat's heart perfusion pressure was increased from 40 to 120 mm Hg. The blocade of nitric oxide production with N^G-monomethyl-l-arginine (Wellcome U.K., 100 mcM) removed autoregulation of coronary vessels (autoregulation gain was negative) completely in the isolated heart, reduced maximum reactive hyperemia coronary flow by 31-36% and respectively reduced the coronary vasodilator reserve by 28.5%. Distensibility of coronary vessels decreased in the average by 32.5% under the influence bloker. The ability of vessels to constrict in response to the perfusion pressure increase was decreased in N^G-monomethyl-l-arginine-treated hearts. After N^G-monomethyl-l-arginine : (a) degree of increase of coronary flow on nitroprusside was similar with control, (b) dependence of developing intravetricular pressure on value of coronary flow is not changed. In conclusion it is noted that maximum changes is coronary flow after blocade was found in earlier period of response of heart vessels to change in perfusion pressure: their rigidity increase, autoregulatory response and also reactive hyperemic coronary flow decreased. In that way, the presented data underline the fact that nitric oxide really play a significant role in the mechanisms of coronary autoregulation.

133

NITRIC OXIDE BUT NOT PEROXYNITRITE RELAXES α-TOXIN PERMEABILIZED SMOOTH MUSCLE OF RAT TAIL ARTERY

A. Soloviev, P. Hellstrand[#] and A. Stefanov
Department of Experimental Therapeutics, Institute of Pharmacology and Toxicology, Academy of Medical Sciences, 14 Eugene Pottier Str., 252057 Kiev, Ukraine and [#]Department Physiology and Neuroscience, Lund University, Solvegatan 19, S-223 62 Lund, Sweden

The purpose of this study was to compare the effects of nitric oxide (NO) and peroxynitrite ($ONOO^-$) on intact (iSM) and α-toxin permeabilized (pSM) smooth muscle (SM) of rat tail artery. It was shown that NO-containing (30 μM) aqueous solution relaxed pSM preactivated with 10^{-6} M Ca^{2+}, indicating that NO decreased Ca^{2+}-sensitivity of myofibrlls. These relaxant responses were not prevented by methylene blue (50 μM), an inhibitor of soluble guanylyl cyclase but significantly decreased by dithioerytritol (5 mM) which maintains SH-groups in reduced state making them uncapable of nitrosylation. NO had not any effect on pSM preconstricted with mycrocystin-LR (10 μM) known as an inhibitor of protein phosphatases. It is important to note that in some cases these NO-induced relaxant responses were preceded by a transient contraction. Externally applied $ONOO^-$ (50 μM) produced a contraction only without following relaxation, suggesting that the constriction component of the response of pSM to NO was due to the conversion of NO in aqueous solution to $ONOO^-$. Neither NO, nor $ONOO^-$ did exibit their actions in Triton X-100 pSM. Both NO and $ONOO^-$ relaxed iVSM in a similar dose-dependent manner. The observed responses to $ONOO^-$ in iSM did not requre the presence of endothelium. It is concluded that Ca^{2+}-desensitizing effect is intrinsic to NO but not for its metabolic derivate, $ONOO^-$.

134

ACUTE (NONGENOMIC) AND LONG-TERM (GENOMIC) EFFECTS OF TESTOSTERONE ON VASORELAXATION IN RAT AORTA

J. N. Stallone and A.Q. Ding
Department of Physiology, Northeastern Ohio Universities College of Medicine, Rootstown, OH 44272, USA

Clinical and experimental data suggest that the gonadal steroid hormones modulate vascular function. Thus, we examined acute (nongenomic) and long-term (genomic) effects of testosterone on vasorelaxation mechanisms in rat thoracic aorta. Aortic rings from male and female Sprague-Dawley rats were prepared for isometric tension recording. Maximal contractile responses to vasopressin (10^{-11}-10^{-6} M) in endothelium-intact aortae were higher in females (4,645±212 mg/mg ring weight) than in males (1,375±222), primarily due to a greater effect of nitric oxide in males (determined by nitric oxide synthase inhibition). Gonadectomy of male rats potentiated contractile responses to vasopressin and eliminated attenuating effects of nitric oxide. Gonadectomy of female rats had no effect on these responses. These effects of testosterone were absent in Testicular-feminized male rats, which lack functional intracellular androgen receptors. In normal male rat aortae precontracted with phenylephrine, acute testosterone (5-300 μM) produced rapid, dose-dependent vasorelaxation via both endothelium-dependent (nitric oxide) and -independent mechanisms. Testosterone produced identical effects in normal female and Testicular-feminized male rat aortae. Endothelium-independent vasorelaxation was selectively attenuated by 4-aminopyridine (5 mM), suggesting involvement of delayed rectifier K^+ channels. Androgen analog experiments revealed that testosterone-induced vasorelaxation is enhanced in polar analogs with lower permeability to the cell membrane. These data demonstrate that testosterone exerts both genomic and nongenomic effects on vasorelaxation mechanisms in rat aorta. (Supported by NIH: HL-47432).

135

IMPAIRED α_1-ADRENOCEPTOR MEDIATED CALCIUM INFLUX IN MESENTERIC RESISTANCE ARTERIES OF THE RAT AFTER MYOCARDIAL INFARCTION

F.R.M.Stassen, M.J.F.F.M. Willemsen, J.G.R. De Mey
Dept. Of Pharmacology, Cardiovascular Research Institute Maastricht, Universiteit Maastricht, PO box 616, Maastricht, the Netherlands.

After myocardial infarction (MI), various neurohumoral mechanisms are activated to maintain systemic perfusion pressure. We evaluated whether the peripheral vasculature adapts to this condition. Myocardial infarction (MI) was induced in male Wistar rats by permanent ligation of the left coronary artery. Five weeks post-MI or sham operation, mesenteric resistance arteries (MrA) were isolated, denuded of endothelium, chemically sympathectomized, depleted of neuropeptides and mounted in a myograph. In the presence of 2.5mM calcium contractile responses to phenylephrine (PHE, 10nM-10μM) were reduced (E_{max} -18%) while responses to 125 mM K^+ with or without 10μM PHE were not modified. Responses to 10μM PHE in the absence of calcium were not altered. Contractile responses to calcium (10μM-10mM) were reduced in the presence of 10μM PHE but were not modified in the presence of 125 mM K^+ +/- 10μM PHE or 1μM PMA. Also the density of [^{3}H]-prazosin binding sites was not reduced in vessels post-MI (3.03±1.40 fmol/μg DNA) compared to sham (2.29±0.21fmol/μg DNA). Thus, the reduced α_1-adrenergic reactivity of MrA post-MI seems to involve primarily an impaired coupling of α_1-adrenoceptors to a calcium-influx pathway.

136

EFFECTS OF DIADENOSINEPOLYPHOSPHATES (APnA'S) ON THE REACTIVITY OF INNERVATED AND NON-INNERVATED RESISTANCE ARTERIES OF THE RAT

M. Steinmetz*, K.H. Rahn*, J.G.R. De Mey
Dept. of Pharmacology, University of Maastricht, P.O. Box 616, 6200 MD Maastricht, The Netherlands; *Dept. of Internal Medicine, University of Münster, Germany

APnA's (n ranging from 3 to 6) have been identified in several tissues (e.g. in the adrenal medulla). Also adenine nucleotides act as sympathetic co-transmitters in arteries. We therefore compared effects of APnA's, ATP, ADP and the stable P2x-purinoceptor agonist $\alpha\beta$-CH_3-ATP in densely innervated mesenteric artery side-branches (MES, ø 200 μm) and non-innervated superior epigastric artery (SEA, ø 300 μm) mounted in a myograph. In both MEA and SEA, all agents induced contraction (rank order of potency: $\alpha\beta$-CH_3-ATP > AP5A ≥ AP6A > AP4A = ATP > ADP > AP3A). In SEA, contractile responses were stable for at least 10 min. In MES, responses were highly transient (103 min). During contraction induced by phenylephrine (10 μM), all agents induced triphasic responses: (a) an initial rapid transient relaxation (2-10 s), (b) an increase in tone to above the level of preconstriction followed by a late sustained relaxation. For all agents the relaxation was more pronounced in MES (60-90%) than in SEA (10-20%). In MES, contractile and relaxing effects of AP5A (10 μM) were not modified by removal of endothelium, acute sympathectomy or depletion of sensory motor nerves but were blunted after exposure to 10 μM PPADS. Thus, in resistance arteries APnA's seem to act primarily on P2x-purinoceptors. In the densely innervated MES their contractile action seems to be counteracted by a direct P2x-receptor mediated relaxation, which could explain their reported biphasic effect on total peripheral resistance.

137

THE MOTILITY ASSAY IN STUDY OF PATHOPHYSIOLOGY OF SMOOTH MUSCLE

NL Stephens and H Jiang
Department of Physiology, University of Manitoba, Winnipeg, MB CANADA R3E 3J7 and Section of Molecular Cardiology, NHLBI, NIH Bethesda, Maryland 20892

While disturbances in contractility of smooth muscle can result from disordered function of contractile and regulatory proteins the motility assay makes it possible to study the molecular motor itself.

In a canine model of "asthma" we reported that maximum velocity of shortening (V_o) of airway smooth muscle (ASM) is significantly increased. We conducted studies to elucidate the biochemical basis of the increased V_o and found that myofibrillar ATPase activity was increased.

Since recent work by Rayment's group suggests that ATPase activity and motility could be associated non-linearly or even dissociated, we tested the hypothesis that changes in actin-myosin motility could be increased (as judged by the motility assay) and exert an additive effect in producing increased V_o. The motility assay consisted in measuring the velocity of translation of chicken gizzard actin filaments by myosin purified from control and "asthmatic" canine airway smooth muscle. V_o for sensitized myosin was 0.868 ± 0.173 SE (n = 58) and control was 0.754 ± 0.189 (n = 60); these means were not significantly different indicating no alteration in contractility at molecular motor level. However we did find a positive dose-response relationship between myosin light chain kinase (MLCK) concentration and V_o as measured by motility assay. We concluded the increased V_o of "asthmatic" airway smooth muscle is likely due to increased degree of phosphorylation of the 20 kDa myosin light chain resulting from increased total MLCK activity that we had also reported.(Supported by grants from the MRC and Inspiraplex, Canada.)

138

NEUROKININ-1(NK-1) RECEPTORS IN THE CEREBROVASCULAR PARASYMPATHETIC NERVES

N.Suzuki, Y.Fukuuchi, A.Koto, Y.Morita, T.Shimizu, M.Takao
Department of Neurology, Keio University, Shinjuku, Tokyo, Japan

Substance P(SP) and vasoactive intestinal polypeptide(VIP) are known to be neurotransmitters in the vasodilatory nerves of the cerebral blood vessels. The two systems containing them, i.e., the sensory and the parasympathetic, respectively, have been elucidated to have extracranial origins and to innervate the cerebral vessels independently. Their relationship or interaction, however, has not been demonstrated. The purpose of this study is to investigate the distribution of neurokinin-1(NK-1) receptors of the cerebral vessels utilizing recently developed NK-1 receptor specific antibody (kindly provided by Dr.R.Shigemoto, Kyoto Univ.), and to explore the relation with the cerebrovascular vasodilatory nerves.

Five male Sprague-Dawley rats were perfused with fixatives and the pial arteries were dissected to be served as whole-mount preparations. Double immunohistochemical techniques for NK-1 receptor and SP or VIP were applied on these preparations.

Numerous NK-1 receptor-like immunoreactivity was noted along the nerve fibers with VIP-like immunoreactivity in all regions of the pial arteries. They consisted of fine, delicate varicose fibers and thick bundles without varicosities. NK-1 receptor-like immunoreactive materials were apparently located on the surface of VIP-positive nerve fibers.

This study demonstrated that VIP containing parasympathetic nerves are equipped with NK-1 receptors in their axonal membranes, which may indicate that the sensory nerves modulate the function of the parasympathetic nerves in the cerebral vessels.

139

IMPAIRED RELAXATION RESPONSES OF WISTAR-KYOTO (WKY) OR SPONTANEOUSLY HYPERTENSIVE (SHR) AORTAE TO NEUTROPHILS (PMNs) FROM SHR IS ONLY ENDOTHELIUM INDEPENDENT.

A.A. Taylor, M.J. Akpaffiong
Center for Experimental Therapeutics, Baylor College of Medicine, One Baylor Plaza, Houston, Texas, 77030, U.S.A

This study examined effects of neutrophils (PMNs) from normotensive (Wistar-Kyoto, WKY) and spontaneously hypertensive (SHR) rats on vascular tone and whether differences in vascular responses to PMNs from WKY and SHR were endothelium-dependent or -independent. PMNs were isolated from peritoneal lavage fluid of WKY and SHR 16 hr after peritoneal instillation of 6% oyster glycogen and reconstituted at $10x10^7$ cells/ml. Thoracic aortic rings from SHR and WKY rats ± endothelium were mounted in organ chambers containing physiologic salt solution at 37°C and gassed with 95% O_2 5% CO_2. Tonic responses of phenylephrine (10^{-6}M) precontracted aortas to PMNs ± indomethacin, nitro-L-arginine (NLA) and 2-phenyl-4,4,5,5-tetramethylimidazoline-1-oxyl-3-oxide (PTIO) were studied. PMNs from SHR rats induced a concentration-dependent relaxation of aortic rings ± endothelium from SHR and WKY rats which was significantly less than that induced by PMNs from WKY rats. Relaxations induced by PMNs from either SHR or WKY on aortic rings from either SHR or WKY rats were not affected by indomethacin, were reversed by NLA and blocked by PTIO. These findings suggest that impaired production of PMN-derived NO and/or EDHF may contribute to the hypertension observed in SHR.

140

ENDOTHELIUM-DEPENDENT HYPERPOLARIZATION IN PORCINE CORONARY ARTERIES WITH REGENERATED ENDOTHELIUM: DECREASED RESPONSE TO SEROTONIN AND INCREASED HYPERPOLARIZATION TO BRADYKININ

C. Thollon, J.P. Bidouard, C. Cambarrat, I. Delescluse, P.M. Vanhoutte, and J.P. Vilaine.
Institut de Recherches Servier, Suresnes, France.

The endothelium-dependent hyperpolarizations induced by serotonin and bradykinin were compared in porcine coronary arteries with native or regenerated endothelium, four weeks after balloon denudation. The transmembrane potential was measured using conventional glass microelectrodes. The experiments were performed in the presence of inhibitors of NO synthase (nitro-L-arginine, L-NA) and cyclooxygenase (indomethacin). Smooth muscle cells from coronary arteries with regenerated endothelium were depolarized in comparison with control arteries. Spontaneous membrane potential oscillations of small amplitude or spikes were observed in some of these arteries but not in normal arteries. The hyperpolarization induced by serotonin (10 µM, in the presence of ketanserin), was significantly lower in coronary arteries with regenerated endothelium than in those with native endothelium. In control coronary arteries an endothelium-dependent hyperpolarization of about 20 mV was obtained with bradykinin (30 nM). In arteries with regenerated endothelium, the hyperpolarization to bradykinin was voltage-dependent, whereby an enhanced hyperpolarization, that could reach -40 mV, could be observed in the most depolarized cells. The changes in membrane potential observed in coronary arteries with regenerated endothelium may contribute to the reduced relaxation to serotonin and the unchanged response to bradykinin that have been described previously.

141

HETEROGENEITY OF EDHF-MEDIATED RELAXATIONS IN SMALL AND LARGE ARTERIES: POSSIBLE ROLE OF THE REDUCTION IN THE CA^{2+} SENSITIVITY OF THE CONTRACTILE APPARATUS BY MEMBRANE HYPERPOLARIZATION

H. Tomioka, M. Fukao*, I. Sakuma, A. Sato, M. Liu, A. Kitabatake and M. Kanno*
Departments of Cardiovascular Medicine and Pharmacology*, Hokkaido University School of Medicine, Sapporo 060, Japan

Heterogeneous distribution of EDHF-mediated relaxations has been reported in several arteries. However, the mechanisms by which EDHF-mediated relaxations are prominent in smaller arteries have not been fully examined. This study was aimed to clarify this point. We measured endothelium-dependent and independent relaxations and hyperpolarizations in the thoracic aorta, the main trunk and the 1st branch of the mesenteric artery in rat. Endothelium-dependent relaxation to acetylcholine in the presence of L-NNA and indomethacin was larger in smaller arteries and was absent in the aorta. In contrast, endothelium-dependent hyperpolarizations were not so much different. Acetylcholine hyperpolarized the membrane potential by 11 mV even in the aorta. Pinacidil produced comparable endothelium-independent hyperpolarization in all of these arteries. However, relaxations by pinacidil were more prominent in smaller arteries. SNP and nifedipine produced relaxations in these arteries to a similar extent.

These results indicate that EDHF-mediated relaxation would be not determined simply by the extent of membrane hyperpolarization, but modulated by another factor such as a difference in the relaxation of Ca^{2+} sensitivity induced by the membrane hyperpolarization of the cell.

142

DIFFERENTIAL EFFECTS OF ISOPRENALINE AND FORSKOLIN ON CYCLIC AMP PRODUCTION IN THE PORCINE CORONARY ARTERY

A.E.Tomlinson, V.G.Wilson
Department of Physiology and Pharmacology, Queen's Medical Centre, Nottingham, UK. NG7 2UH.

Beta-adrenoceptor-mediated vascular relaxation is generally accepted to involve G-protein-dependent stimulation of adenylyl cyclase and an associated increase in cyclic AMP. However in the bovine coronary artery equieffective dilator concentrations of forskolin and isoprenaline produced different levels of cyclic AMP (Vesgna RVK et al. Can J Physiol Pharmacol 1983; 61: 1202-1205). Using a [3H]-adenine pre-labelling assay for measurement of cyclic AMP we have examined the effect of these two dilators in the porcine coronary artery.

Isoprenaline (0.5µM) and forskolin (0.5µM) relaxed U46619-induced contractions of the porcine coronary artery by 90% and elevated [3H]-cyclic AMP accumulation by 40-50% (table 1). The phosphodiesterase inhibitor rolipram (10µM) produced a marked increase (80%) in the level of cyclic AMP (table 1) but differentially potentiated forskolin-induced (2-fold) and isoprenaline-induced (4-fold) elevation of cyclic AMP (table 1).

Table 1: % Conversion of [3H]-adenine to [3H]-cyclic AMP in the porcine coronary artery. (n=7)

	Control	10µM rolipram
Basal	0.10 ± 0.01	0.18 ± 0.03
0.5µM forskolin	0.15 ± 0.03	0.33 ± 0.05 *
0.5µM isoprenaline	0.14 ± 0.02	0.55 ± 0.07 *

* indicates significant difference from control (unpaired Student's t-test, $P \leq 0.05$).

These results raise the possibility that responses involved in the beta-adrenoceptor activation and direct activation of adenylyl cyclase to elevate cyclic AMP are mediated in different cellular compartments.

143

FLOW-MEDIATED ARTERIAL REMODELING IN RAT MESENTERIC VASCULATURE

D.A. Tulis, J.L. Unthank*, R.L. Prewitt
Department of Physiology, Eastern Virginia Medical School, Norfolk, Virginia, 23501, and *Indiana University Medical Center, Indianapolis, Indiana, 46202 USA

This study was designed to characterize structural adaptations of male Wistar rat small mesenteric arteries exposed to elevated blood flow in vivo for 1, 3, or 7 days. A series of arterial ligations caused blood flow and calculated wall shear rate to approximately double in the ileal artery feeding the flow-restricted section. Neither mean carotid nor local mesenteric arterial pressures changed significantly pre- to post-ligation. Significant luminal expansion and medial wall hypertrophy occurred in the feeding ileal and second-order branch arteries in a time-dependent fashion between 1 and 7 days of elevated flow when compared to same animal control-flow vessels. Wall thickness to lumen diameter ratios did not change in any vessel at any time. These results suggest circumferential wall stress is held constant and these morphological changes represent shear stress-induced structural remodeling.

Immunostaining for proliferating cell nuclear antigen and nuclear profile analyses indicate that both medial smooth muscle cell and intimal endothelial cell hyperplasia contribute to shear stress-induced alterations in the vessel wall. Immunostaining for endothelial nitric oxide synthase suggests its upregulation in response to elevated flow at all time points. In situ hybridization reveals significantly increased mRNA for platelet-derived growth factor-A chain in the media after exposure to flow for 24 hours. These findings suggest shear stress-stimulated vasodilation in vivo involves nitric oxide while vessel wall growth is related to increased expression of platelet-derived growth factor-A chain.

144

THE RELAXATION INDUCED BY NICOTINE IN THE RAT ISOLATED RENAL ARTERY

S. Emre, I. Ay, M. Tuncer
Department of Pharmacology, University of Hacettepe, 06100, Ankara, Turkey

The mechanism of nicotine-induced relaxation was investigated in the rat isolated renal artery.

Wistar rats of both sexes were anesthetized, left renal arteries were removed and cut into rings. Two fine, steel pins were introduced through the lumen of vascular segments and they were prepared for isometric recording in organ bath containing Krebs-Henseleit solution (37^{0}C) bubbled with a gas mixture (95% O_2 and 5% CO_2).

Nicotine (10^{-3} M) produced a relaxation when preparations were precontracted by phenylephrine (3×10^{-6} M). Nicotine-induced relaxation was 28.96±3.36% of phenylephrine contraction and was not affected by atropine (10^{-5} M), guanethidine (10^{-5} M), hexamethonium (10^{-4} M), indomethacine (10^{-5} M), N^G-nitro-L-arginine (10^{-4} M), methylene blue (10^{-5} M), glibenclamide (10^{-5} M), quinacrine (3×10^{-5} M), tetrodotoxin (10^{-6} M), capsaicin (10^{-6} M), tetraethylammonium (10^{-3} M), 4-amino-pyridine (10^{-3} M) and ouabain (10^{-6} M), (n=6, Mann Whitney U test). Neither a calcium antagonizing effect of nicotine was observed.

These results suggest that nicotine at the concentration used causes a relaxation which is not mediated by the stimulation of nicotinic receptors, release of nitric oxide, prostanoids, endothelium-derived hyperpolarizing factor and tachykinin neuromediators, in the rat renal artery.

145

THE FACTORS WHICH ARE RESPONSIBLE FOR ACETYLCHOLINE-INDUCED DILATATION OF RAT RENAL VASCULATURE

M. Tuncer, I. Ay
Department of Pharmacology, University of Hacettepe, 06100, Ankara, Turkey

We examined the mechanism of acetylcholine-induced dilatation in the isolated perfused rat kidneys.

Wistar rats of both sexes were anesthetized with ether and kidneys were isolated and perfused via renal artery. Optimal perfusion pressure was found to be 70-90 mmHg and optimal flow rate was 8-10 ml/min.

In control experiments acetylcholine caused dose-dependent dilatation. The maximum dilatation was 65.38±4.05% of maximum phenylephrine constriction. Atropine (10^{-6} M), hexamethonium (10^{-4} M), indomethacin (10^{-5} M), N^G-nitro-L-arginine (10^{-4} M), glibenclamide (10^{-5} M), 4-amino-pyridine (10^{-3} M), attenuated the acetylcholine-induced dilatation significantly ($p<0.05$, n=6, ANOVA). Tetraethylammonium (10^{-3} M), ouabain (10^{-6} M) and quinacrine ($3\text{x}10^{-6}$ M) did not change the dilatation. On the other hand, methylene blue (10^{-5} M), tetrodotoxin (10^{-6} M) and capsaicin (10^{-6} M) caused a significant inhibition in acetylcholine-induced dilatation ($p<0.01$, n=6, ANOVA).

These results suggest that acetylcholine-induced dilatation may occur via factors released from endothelium and/or presynaptic nerve endings and act through soluble guanylate cyclase and both ATP-sensitive and voltage-dependent potassium channels in the isolated perfused rat kidney.

146

NICOTINE-INDUCED VASODILATATION IN THE ISOLATED PERFUSED RAT KIDNEY

M. Tuncer, I. Ay
Department of Pharmacology, University of Hacettepe, 06100, Ankara, Turkey

The aim of this study was to investigate the mechanism of nicotine-induced vasodilatation in isolated perfused rat kidney.

Wistar rats of both sexes were anesthetized with ether and kidneys isolated and perfused via renal artery under a constant flow rate using a peristaltic pump. Optimal perfusion pressure was found to be 70-90 mmHg and optimal flow rate was 8-10 ml/min.

Nicotine (100µg/0.1 ml) produced a constriction which was 8.39±0.7% of maximum phenylephrine response (n=4). When preparations were preconstricted by phenylephrine ($3\text{x}10^{-6}$ M), nicotine (100 µg/0.1 ml) caused a dilatation which was 24.97±3.27 % of maximum phenylephrine constriction (n=5). Nicotine-induced dilatation was resistant to 4-amino-pyridine (10^{-3} M), atropine (10^{-6} M), capsaicin (10^{-6} M), glibenclamide (10^{-5} M), guanethidine (10^{-5} M), hexamethonium (10^{-4} M), indomethacin (10^{-5} M), methylene blue (10^{-5} M), N^G-nitro-L-arginine (10^{-4} M), ouabain (10^{-6} M), quinacrine ($3\text{x}10^{-6}$ M), tetraethylammonium (10^{-3} M) and tetrodotoxin (10^{-6} M) (n=5, Mann Whitney U test).

These results suggested that nicotine-induced dilatation at the dose of 100 µg/0.1 ml was not due to nitric oxide released from endothelium, smooth muscle or nitrergic nerves, endothelium-derived hyperpolarizing factor, prostanoids and factors released from afferent nerve endings and stimulation of nicotinic receptors in the isolated perfused rat kidney.

147

THE THERMO-INDUCED MECHANICAL REACTIONS OF AORTA IN THE CASES OF EXPERIMENTAL ATHEROGENESIS

V.O. Uzhvan, V.I. Mirutenko, M.F. Shuba
Biophysical Laboratory, Kyiv Taras Shevchenko University, Volodymyrska st. 64, 252017 Kyiv, Ukraine

The thermo-induced mechanical reactions of aorta isolated strips from guinea pigs and rabbits in experimental atherogenesis were studied in isometric regimen. Experimental animals had been fed an atherogenic diet (guinea pigs during 4 months; rabbits during 2 months).

Preparations were stretched slowly on 40% of their initial length and were kept in the Krebs solution during 1 hr. The isolated longitudinal and transverse strips were influenced by temperature from 20°C to 40°C. It was found that thermo-sensitive mechanical reactions of intercellular connective tissue matrix of aorta preparations from the experimental animals decreased for 40-60% during the atherogenesis process in comparison with control animals. The mechanical tension of aorta strips by the action of noradrenaline (10^{-5} M) for the experimental animals was less than in control ones. At the same time, the increase of stiffness was equal in both cases by the actions of noradrenaline. Relaxation of aorta strips from experimental animals slows down considerably after every repeated effect of temperature. The action of papaverine completely removed the stiffness and only partly reduced the mechanical tension.

It is suggested that the papaverine-insensitive tension is non-actomyosin in its nature and is connected with the thermo-induced mechanical reactions of intercellular connective tissue matrix.

148

INFLUENCE OF CYTOCHROME P450 INHIBITORS ON EDHF- AND CROMAKALIM-INDUCED RELAXATIONS IN RAT MAIN MESENTERIC ARTERIES

J. Van de Voorde, B. Vanheel
Department of Physiology and Physiopathology, University of Gent, De Pintelaan 185, B-9000 Gent, Belgium.

In several blood vessels, endothelium-dependent vasorelaxation is in part mediated by an endothelium-derived hyperpolarizing factor (EDHF), the nature of which is as yet unknown. However, some evidence suggests that EDHF might be a cytochrome P450-dependent mono-oxygenase metabolite of arachidonic acid. Using isometric tension measurements on rat main mesenteric arteries, the influence of four structurally and mechanistically different cytochrome P450 inhibitors (proadifen, miconazole, 1-amino-benzotriazole, 17-octadecynoic acid) was investigated on relaxations elicited by EDHF, assessed as the nitro-L-arginine resistant component of acetylcholine-induced relaxation, and on relaxations provoked by the endothelium-independent potassium channel opener cromakalim. Proadifen (30 μM) inhibited the EDHF- as well as the cromakalim-induced relaxation, but not that elicited by nitroprusside. Also miconazole (30 μM) inhibited both the EDHF and the cromakalim-induced relaxation. On the other hand, 17-octadecynoic acid (5 μM) had no influence and 1-aminobenzotriazole (1 mM) even potentiated EDHF- and cromakalim-induced relaxations. We conclude that the EDHF, released from the rat mesenteric artery by acetylcholine, is unlikely a cytochrome P450-dependent mono-oxygenase metabolite of arachidonic acid and that proadifen and miconazole interfere with the action of cromakalim.

149

INFLUENCE OF CYTOCHROME P450 INHIBITORS ON HYPERPOLARIZATION AND K^+ CURRENT OF VASCULAR SMOOTH MUSCLE

B. Vanheel, P. Calders, J. Van de Voorde
Department of Physiology and Physiopathology, University of Gent, De Pintelaan 185, B–9000 Gent, Belgium.

The influence of five different inhibitors of cytochrome P450 was tested on the acetylcholine (1 μM)–induced endothelium–dependent hyper–polarization and on the levcromakalim (300 nM)–induced hyper–polarization of smooth muscle from the rat main mesenteric artery. The cytochrome P450 inhibitor proadifen (30 μM) completely and reversibly inhibited the acetylcholine–induced hyperpolarization. However, proadifen also completely inhibited endothelium–independent hyperpolarization by levcromakalim. In addition, preliminary experiments on isolated smooth muscle cells from the rat aorta showed that proadifen (15 and 30 μM) reversibly depressed whole cell outward K^+ current both in the presence and absence of external Ca^{2+}. The imidazole antimycotics clotrimazole (30 μM) and miconazole (100 μM) decreased but did not abolish the acetylcholine–induced hyperpolarization of mesenteric artery strips. These substances completely inhibited levcromakalim–induced hyperpolarization. The suicide substrate inhibitors 17–octadecynoic acid (5 μM) and 1–aminobenzotriazole (2 mM) did neither influence endothelium–dependent nor endothelium–independent hyperpolarization. These results do not support the view that the cytochrome P450 dependent metabolism of arachidonic acid is involved in the acetylcholine–induced endothelium–dependent hyperpolarization in the rat mesenteric artery.

150

17-β ESTRADIOL IMPLICATION IN VASODILATATION

Y. Vedernikov, M. Belfort, G. Saade, R.Garfield.
Department of Obstetrics and Gynecology, University of Texas Medical Branch, Galveston, TX 77555, USA

The beneficial effect of 17-β estradiol on the cardiovascular system is linked to its effect on lipoprotein metabolism, neuromediators, Ca^{++} and the L-arginine-nitric-oxide pathway. In omental artery rings from nonpregnant, normotensive pregnant and preeclamptic patients estradiol decreased tension induced by KC, 60 mM in the presence of phentolamine (10^{-6} M), pD_2~ 5.2. Inhibition by erstradiol of U 46619-induced contraction was counteracted by indomethacin (10^{-5} M), but not by Nω-nitro-L-arginine (10^{-4} M). Relaxation of KCl-contracted omental artery rings by substance P (10^{-9} M) (without indomethacin) was higher in pregnant compared to nonpregnant and preeclamptic vessels. Estradiol (10^{-5} M) in the presence of phentolamine (10^{-6} M) and ropranolol (10^{-6} M), inhibited calcium concentration-dependent contractions equally in all vessels, while response to norepinephrine (in the presence of propranolol (10^{-6} M) and hydrocortisone ($3x10^{-6}$ M) was inhibited in the vessels from nonpregnant patients only. In aortic rings of ovariectomized rats estradiol (10 μg/rat/day for 10 days) did not effect endothelium-dependent relaxation by acetylcholine, slightly counteracted inhibition of the response induced by Nω-nitro-L-arginine and did not influence relaxation by SIN-1 in phenylephrine contracted rings. The beneficial effect of estradiol on the cardiovascular system may not be due to the activation of L-arginine-nitric oxide pathway, but rather to its effect on cycloxygenase and calcium translocation through voltage-dependent calcium channels.

151

AN IN VITRO MODEL OF SELECTIVE ENDOTHELIAL DYSFUNCTION

N. Villeneuve, V. Marteau, C. Jacquemin, C. Petit, A. Pillon, P.M. Vanhoutte, and J.P. Vilaine
Institut de Recherches Servier, 11 rue des Moulineaux 92150 Suresnes, France.

The vascular reactivity of porcine coronary arteries was studied after a prolonged incubation in culture medium in conventional organ chambers. Coronary artery rings were incubated at 37°C in culture medium (MEM) with antibiotics supplement for 20 to 22 hours. Silver nitrate staining confirmed the presence of endothelial cells with a normal morphology in these incubated rings.

After 22 hours of incubation, the contractile responses of smooth muscle cells were normal but the endothelium-dependent relaxations to serotonin, in the presence of ketanserin and indomethacin, were decreased. Nevertheless, the endothelium-dependent relaxations to bradykinin, as well as the endothelium-independent relaxations to a nitric oxide donor were maintained. Under these conditions, the basal production of cGMP was also decreased markedly. L-arginine supplementation of the culture medium had no effect on the endothelial dysfunction. These findings indicate that a prolonged incubation of porcine coronary arteries in culture medium does not produce disruption of vascular endothelial cells, but impairs the endothelium-dependent relaxations mediated by Gi proteins as observed in various experimental chronic models. This could represent a convenient *in vitro* model for the study of the mechanism underlying the selective endothelial dysfunction and for the research of a therapeutic strategy.

152

PRESSURE-INDUCED MYOGENIC RESPONSES IN CEREBRAL RESISTANCE ARTERIES ISOLATED FROM TRANSGENIC (mREN-2)27 HYPERTENSIVE RATS.

S.J.Wallis, S.M. Gardiner, W.R. Dunn.
Department of Physiology and Pharmacology, Queen's Medical Centre, Nottingham, NG7 2UH, UK.

We have previously shown that the middle cerebral artery (MCA) isolated from genetically hypertensive Brattleboro rats, displays enhanced pressure-induced myogenic responses, compared to vessels from normotensive controls (Dunn & Wallis, J.Vasc.Res. 1996; 33 (Suppl. 2): 16). In the present study we have examined the pressure-induced myogenic responses of the MCA, isolated from hypertensive transgenic (TG) rats expressing the mouse Ren-2 gene (TGR(mRen-2)27), in comparison with normotensive Sprague Dawley (SD) control rats. Arteries from TG rats (MAP 155±4mmHg, n=13) and SD rats (MAP 112±5mmHg, n=13), were set up in a Halpern pressure myograph and diameter was determined in calcium-containing (1.6mmol/L) physiological salt solution (PSS), through the pressure range 10-170mmHg, in stepwise increments of 20mmHg. This was repeated in calcium-free PSS (containing 0.5mmol/L EGTA), to determine the passive pressure-diameter relationship. At 10mmHg, vessels from TG rats had a greater degree of intrinsic tone, than arteries from SD rats (% induced tone, TG: 17.4±3.5% vs. SD: 2.1±1.7% $p<0.05$ Student's t-t est). However, there was no significant difference in active pressure-induced myogenic tone in the MCA isolated from TG and SD rats at pressures greater than 10mmHg (e.g. at 90mmHg % induced tone, TG: 23.9±3.6% vs. SD: 25.4±3.7%). Thus, in contrast to genetically hypertensive Brattleboro rats, pressure-induced myogenic responses are not enhanced in cerebral resistance arteries isolated from TG hypertensive rats, at physiologically relevant pressures.

SJ Wallis is supported by a MRC studentship.

153

KINETICS OF REACTIVE HYPEREMIA: PEAK POSTISCHEMIC VASODILATION IS RELATED TO FOREARM COMPOSITION IN HEALTHY SUBJECTS.

T.C. Wascher, *R. Stollberger, *R. Pammer, S. Wallner, H. Toplak
Deptartment of Internal Medicine and *Magnetic Resonance Institute, University of Graz, 8036 Graz, Austria

Postischemic reactive hyperemia is frequently used to determine unaltered functional reactivity of vascular beds by means of vascular reserve. This process, however, is dynamic and current literature reveals a wide diversion of measured values and time points. Aim of the present study was to determine kinetics of reactive hyperemia in healthy subjects in relation to forearm composition.

Reactive hyperemia (ml/min/100ml forearm) was measured in 8 healthy volunteers (4 male, 4 female, age 18-35 years, BMI 18-25 kg/m^2) by venous occlusion plethysmography after 1, 2, and 5 minutes of global ischemia (every 10" for 60"). Forearm composition was determined by serial magnetic resonance imaging with computed signal analysis. Values are mean ± SD, correlation by Pearson Matrix.

Resting blood flow was 2.4±1.2 ml/min/100ml. Ischemia dose dependently ($p<0.02$) increased peak RH (observed at 10") and $t_{1/2}$ of reactive hyperemia. Whereas $t_{1/2}$ was independent of forearm composition, peak values after 2 (15.5±4.4 ml/min/100ml, r=0.747, $p<0.033$) and 5 (30.8±11.7 ml/min/100ml, r=0.804, $p<0.016$) minutes of ischemia strongly correlated to relative forearm muscle mass. 1 minute peak flow and resting flow were independent of forearm composition.

In conclusion, our data demonstrate that forearm muscle mass determines the early peak of reactive hyperemia but not duration in healthy subjects.

154

CALCIUM-DEPENDENT ACTIVATION OF CHLORIDE CURRENT IN HUMAN AORTIC ENDOTHELIAL CELLS

Makino Watanabe and Rikuo Ochi
Department of Physiology, Juntendo University School of Medicine, 2-1-1 Hongo, Bunkyo-ku, Tokyo 113, Japan

In vascular endothelial cells Cl^- currents are activated by several vasoactive agonists associated with an increase in $[Ca^{2+}]_i$ and by hypoosmotic cell-swelling. We examined the effects of $[Ca^{2+}]_i$ to activation of Cl^- currents by applying Ca^{2+} intracellularly with diffusion from pipette solutions and utilizing Ca^{2+} ionophore. Whole-cell membrane currents were recorded by patch clamp technique, and $[Ca^{2+}]_i$ was measured simultaneously by Fura-2 fluorometry. Intracellular Ca^{2+} application by break-in of Ca^{2+} buffer solutions produced outward-going Cl^- currents. The delay between the rise of $[Ca^{2+}]_i$ and the increase of Cl^- currents was 1 to 2 minutes. At isoosmotic condition (285 mOsm), intracellular diffusion of Ca^{2+} buffer induced Cl^- conductance of 0.75 ± 0.17 nS/pF (n=16, mean ± S.E.) at pCa7.5, 1.12 ± 0.20 nS/pF(n=8) at pCa 6 and 3.33 ± 0.49 nS/pF (n=17) at pCa 5. When the hypotonic 265 mOsm pipette solutions were used, the Cl^- conductance increase was negligible (0.06 ± 0.03 nS/pF, n=4) at pCa 7.5, but was remarkable (0.77 ± 0.22 nS/pF, n=7) at pCa5. Application of ionomycin (10 μM) in the presence of 190 mOsm Ca^{2+}-free pipette solution containing 1 mM EGTA and in the presence of 1.8 mM Ca^{2+} in the superfusate, produced a rapid rise of $[Ca^{2+}]_i$ and a increase of the Cl^- current with a relatively short delay of 10-15 sec. These results indicate that there exist Ca^{2+}-activated as well as volume-activated Cl^- channels in endothelial cells and that the Ca^{2+} dependent activation is not entirely due to direct binding of Ca^{2+} to the Cl^- channels.

155

ACETYLCHOLINE-INDUCED K^+-CURRENTS IN SMOOTH MUSCLE CELLS OF INTACT RAT SMALL ARTERIES

T. Weidelt, W. Boldt, F. Markwardt
J.B. Inst. for Physiology, M.L. University, D-06097 Halle, Germany

The mechanism of the sustained acetylcholine-induced endothelium-dependent hyperpolarization (EDH) in intact rat small mesenteric arteries prestimulated with noradrenaline (10^{-6} M) was investigated by means of the single microelectrode voltage clamp method.
The increase of the mean input resistance R_{inp} of the clamped vascular smooth muscle from 120 MΩ under control conditions to 440 MΩ after application of K^+-channel blocking drugs and the linear dependence of the monoexponential time course of voltage relaxation after injection of hyperpolarizing currents on R_{inp} argue against a coupling between the vascular smooth muscle cells (VSMCs).
Sustained (> 5 min) application of ACh (10^{-5} M) hyperpolarized the VSMCs by induction of a hyperpolarizing current. This effect was completely blocked by the inhibitor of the nitric oxide (NO) synthase L-NAME (10^{-3} M) but not by the inhibitor of the soluble guanylate cyclase (sGCl), methylene blue (MB, 10^{-4} M). Application of the NO-donor sodium nitroprusside (SNP, 10^{-6} M) for more than 5 min mimicked the induction of the endothelium-dependent hyperpolarizing current in vessels with destroyed endothelium. This effect of SNP could also not be blocked by MB. Only the combined administration of Glb and CTX blocked the SNP-induced current completely. Our results suggest that in rat small mesenteric artery, ACh hyperpolarizes the VSMCs tonically by activating both ATP- and Ca^{2+}-dependent K^+-currents only via release of NO from the endothelium without need for activation of the sGCl.

156

DIMETHYLSULFOXIDE ATTENUATES THE PRESSOR RESPONSE TO VASOPRESSIN IN THE RABBIT HEART

Margaret T. Weis
Philadelphia College of Pharmacy, Philadelphia PA 19104, U.S.A.

Dimethylsulfoxide has been reported to interfere with vasopressin action in various tissues. These studies arose from the observation that the response to sequential doses of vasopressin is progressively reduced in the presence of dimethylsulfoxide. Four bolus injections (100ng) of vasopressin were administered to Langendorff-perfused rabbit hearts at 15 min intervals. Five minutes after the first dose, dimethylsulfoxide infusion (0.022%) was begun, and continued throughout the experiment. Responses to 4th dose versus 1st dose of vasopressin are shown (*=p<0.05 *vs.* control):

Parameter	Control (n=6)	Experimental (n=6)
Duration	0.78 ± 0.08	0.33 ± 0.06*
Magnitude	0.85 ± 0.05	0.39 ± 0.08*
Rate of rise	0.88 ± 0.06	0.32 ± 0.06*
Rate of fall	0.87 ± 0.12	0.70 ± 0.30
AUC	0.67 ± 0.10	0.24 ± 0.07*

Vasopressin-stimulated 6-keto-$PGF_{1\alpha}$ synthesis was unaffected, suggesting that dimethylsulfoxide does not interfere with V_{1a} receptor function. The effect of dimethylsulfoxide was not reversed by a 30 minute washout. Angiotensin II-mediated vasoconstriction declined from 30 ± 16 to 15 ± 4 mm Hg in the absence and from 32 ± 14 to 31 ± 13 mm Hg in the presence of dimethylsulfoxide, suggesting that the effect is specific for vasopressin. In the presence of dimethylsulfone, maximal pressor resonse to the 4th dose of vasopressin was 92±6% of the response to the 1st dose, indicating that the effect is specific for dimethylsulfoxide. Nitric oxide synthase inhibition restored the duration of the response and the area under the pressor response curve to control values. Supported by NIH (HL-48204).

157

DISSOCIATION OF CYCLIC GMP LEVELS FROM NITRIC OXIDE-INDUCED DECREASE OF INTRACELLULAR CALCIUM AND RELAXATION IN RABBIT AORTIC SMOOTH MUSCLE

R.M. Weisbrod, M. C. Griswold and R.A. Cohen
Vascular Biology Unit, Boston Medical Center, Boston, MA 02118, USA

A decrease in the concentration of intracellular free calcium (Ca^{2+}_i) in vascular smooth muscle via an increase in cyclic GMP and activation of cyclic GMP-dependent protein kinase (PKG) is thought to be the principle mechanism by which nitric oxide (NO) causes relaxation. Our purpose was to determine the role of cyclic GMP in mediating the actions of NO (10^{-10}-10^{-6}M) in rabbit aortic rings and smooth muscle in primary culture with the guanylate cyclase inhibitor, H-[1,2,4] oxadiazolo[4,3-a] quinoxallin-1-one (ODQ, 10µM), the PKG inhibitor, Rp-8-bromo-cyclic GMPs (Rp), the PKG activator, 8-(4-chlorophenylthio)-cyclic GMP (CPT), and the phosphodiesterase inhibitor, zaprinast. Fura-2 was used to measure Ca^{2+}_i and divalent cation influx (as estimated by Mn^{2+} quenching of fura-2). Cyclic GMP was assessed with immunoassay. Decreases in Ca^{2+}_i to NO were unaffected by zaprinast, despite the fact that cyclic GMP was increased up to 20-fold. ODQ significantly inhibited the decrease in Ca^{2+}_i and relaxation caused by lower concentrations of NO (<0.1 µM), but had less or no effect on higher concentrations despite abolishing increases in cyclic GMP. The inhibition by NO (1 µM) of agonist-induced Mn^{2+} influx was unaffected by ODQ. Although Rp completely blocked the inhibition of Mn^{2+} influx caused by CPT, it had no effect on the inhibition of cation influx caused by NO. These data indicate that a significant dissociation exists between cyclic GMP levels and decreases in Ca^{2+}_i and relaxation caused by NO (< 0.1 µM). At concentrations greater than 0.1 µM, NO may act independently of a rise in cyclic GMP to reduce Ca^{2+}_i and cause relaxation.

158

A ROLE FOR ENDOTHELIN AND A PROSTANOID IN ODQ-INDUCED CONTRACTIONS OF THE PORCINE ISOLATED SPLENIC ARTERY

V.G. Wilson, T.Y. Lot, A. Tambyraja.
Department of Physiology & Pharmacology, Queen's Medical Centre, Nottingham, NG7 2UH, UK

Nitric oxide (NO) synthase inhibitors produce endothelium-dependent contractions of the porcine isolated splenic artery (Lot T et al. J Physiol 1995; 487: 82P). In the present study we have examined whether 1H-[1,2,4]oxadiazolo[4,3,-a]quinoxalin-1-one (ODQ), a selective inhibitor of soluble guanylyl cyclase, produces similar responses.

Segments (5mm) of the porcine isolated splenic artery were prepared for isometric tension recording. In endothelium-denuded segments, sodium nitroprusside (1µM)-induced relaxations (>90%) of U46619-induced contractions were abolished by 1µM ODQ. ODQ (1µM) caused a contraction of endothelium-intact segments (21.1±2.7% of the 60mM KCl response, n=10) but not in endothelium-denuded segments (< 2% of the 60mM KCl response, n=5). The ET_A/ET_B receptor antagonist, PD-145065, and the TXA_2/PGH_2 receptor antagonist, vapiprost, inhibited (* p < 0.05, Student's unpaired t-test) ODQ-induced contractions of endothelium-intact segments (Table 1).

Table 1: The effect of PD 145065 (10µM) and Vapiprost (1µM) against ODQ-induced contractions (n=10).

Control	PD-145650	Control	Vapiprost
84.7±4.4	59.6±6.7*	95.4±2.1	66.7±5.7*

Contractions are shown as a percentage of the sustained response prior to the addition of the receptor antagonist.

Thus, blockade of soluble guanylyl cyclase in the porcine splenic isolated artery mimics the effect of inhibition of NO synthase, resulting in endothelium-dependent contractions mediated by endothelin and a prostanoid.

Author Index